RECOMME.

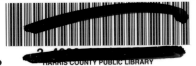

"Every individual who takes care of kids should own this book—parents, teachers, babysitters, and more. The book provides expert guidance and explains complex topics in an understandable and fun way."
—Ann Chen Wu, M.D., F.A.A.P., Professor of Pediatrics at Harvard Medical School

"Dr. Jung has a gift for memorable one-liners which help parents quickly grasp their child's illness, but his book also offers an in-depth, masters-level course for parents who want to truly understand the biology of many common pediatric problems."
—Chris Straughn, M.D., F.A.A.P., Founding Partner of Forest Lane Pediatrics in Dallas, TX

"Dr. Jung's book is very thorough and easy to read. It is totally consistent with what I tell my patients. It's an essential reference for every parent—a must have!"
—Ronald Vilela, M.D., Professor of Pediatric ENT at Texas Children's Hospital

"What a wonderful resource for parents! Dr. Jung is a gifted and experienced pediatrician, and this book can help any parent navigate the often stressful landscape of caring for a sick child."
—Suny Liaw, M.D., F.A.A.P., Professor of Pediatrics at Harvard Medical School

"This book will help parents understand the mechanisms of common illnesses in young children. I think this will provide parents with calm confidence in the face of illness."
—Elizabeth Patterson, mother of two

"This is exactly the kind of highly informative and practical guide that all parents should have on hand to reference common pediatric illnesses. Finally, someone has put together an easy-to-read, but thorough manual that parents can apply to their daily life."
—Edward Lee, M.D., Professor of Pediatric Plastic Surgery at Texas Children's Hospital

Hatherleigh Press is committed to preserving and protecting the natural resources of the earth. Environmentally responsible and sustainable practices are embraced within the company's mission statement.

Visit us at www.hatherleighpress.com and register online for free offers, discounts, special events, and more.

**What to Know Before Seeing Your Pediatrician**
Text copyright © 2015 Peter Jung, M.D.

Library of Congress Cataloging-in-Publication Data is available upon request.
ISBN 978-1-57826-606-7

All Hatherleigh Press titles are available for bulk purchase, special promotions, and premiums. For information about reselling and special purchase opportunities, please call 1-800-528-2550 and ask for the Special Sales Manager.

Cover and Interior Design by Carolyn Kasper

10 9 8 7 6 5 4 3 2 1
Printed in the United States

# What to Know Before Seeing Your Pediatrician

## An Illustrated Guide for Parents

Peter Jung, M.D.

Illustrated by Becky Kim

# Dedication

*This book is dedicated to my family and to all the children who have taught me how to become a better pediatrician.*

—Peter Jung

*To my loving and supportive husband and family, whose unwavering belief in me is the reason why I've accomplished as much as I have. I love you.*

—Becky Kim

# Contents

# Introduction

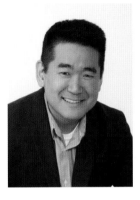

I HAVE ALWAYS believed that an essential role of a pediatrician is being a good educator. Equipping parents with a solid understanding of colds, fevers, and germs can help reduce anxiety and prevent unnecessary visits to the doctor. Over the years, I have come up with some catchphrases and analogies that I commonly employ to help moms and dads understand what is going on with their child. I have also found that a quick drawing on the paper of the exam table helps to drive the point home.

I quickly realized that even a simple illustration can be a powerful tool in explaining a child's illness to their parents. I saw parents taking home my rudimentary drawings to share with their spouses; this gave me the idea to create a picture book to help parents better understand the basics of pediatrics. Luckily, I found a graphics design whiz who was able to transfer the ideas in my brain onto paper—with illustrations far superior to my own!

Each picture in this book is paired with a bit of pediatric wisdom I've gained over the past decade as a practicing doctor. This book is not intended as a comprehensive guide to every illness that your child can encounter, nor is it meant to be a quick reference guide. Rather, it is to be read sequentially, each chapter building upon the next, to provide you with a solid understanding of what happens in the body of a sick child.

My goal is to enable all moms and dads who read this book to get more out of each visit and conversation with their doctor. I hope that by better understanding what is going on in your child's body, you will feel more at ease the next time they come down with a fever or cough.

—Peter Y. Jung, M.D., F.A.A.P.

# Goals

A T THE end of this book, you should be able to fulfill several goals:

**Goal 1**: Understand the difference between bacteria and viruses, and know when antibiotics are necessary.

**Goal 2**: Understand that identifying the source of a fever is far more important than the degree of a fever.

**Goal 3**: Understand the importance of vaccines and how they work.

**Goal 4**: Understand what colds are and how they lead to inflammatory and clogging complications.

**Goal 5**: Understand how ear infections form and how they can be treated.

**Goal 6**: Understand other complications that can be triggered by the common cold.

**Goal 7**: Understand how to prevent dehydration in a child with gastroenteritis.

**Goal 8**: Understand when a child should return to school after an illness.

# Chapter 1

# GERMS

ANY DISCUSSION about a sick child must begin with understanding the basics of germs. There are two major groups of germs that typically infect healthy children: **bacteria** and **viruses**. Fungi and parasites can also lead to infection, but these groups are far less common, and not relevant to this general discussion.

Identifying the key differences between bacteria and viruses will help parents to understand when antibiotics are necessary, and when they are not. Antibiotics can trigger unwanted side effects such as diarrhea and allergic reactions. Thus, it is important to only use antibiotics when they are truly needed. This in turn helps parents to know when a child can be monitored at home, as opposed to when they need to be seen at the doctor's office.

There are many different classes of antibiotics. Choosing the right one is dependent on what type of bacteria is suspected and where in the body the infection is occurring.

# BACTERIA VS. VIRUS

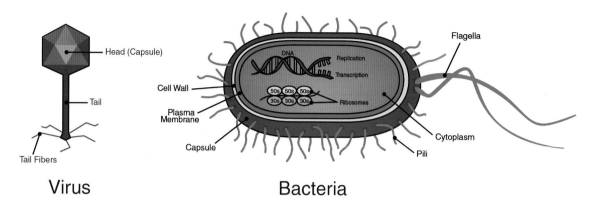

**Virus**

**Bacteria**

The two major groups of germs that make children sick are bacteria and viruses.

The illustration above demonstrates the significant difference in complexity between a virus and a bacterial cell. The picture is not drawn to scale; typical bacteria are generally 10 times bigger than typical viruses. Bacteria also have many organelles and cellular components that are not present in viruses.

This is important to understand, as antibiotics work by attacking different sections of a bacterial cell that simply do not exist in a virus. In other words, antibiotics work on bacteria, but do absolutely nothing against a virus. **This is why antibiotics should never be prescribed for a child who is sick from a virus—it will not help!**

And, as viruses are by far the most common source of illness, most infections do not require antibiotics.

But the word ***antibiotics*** itself can be confusing. Sometimes the term "antibiotics" is used (correctly) to describe a medication that treats viruses or fungi; however, it is more precise to refer to these medications as antivirals or antifungals, respectively. For the purposes of this book, ***antibiotics*** will refer to antibacterial medications, which are only used to treat bacterial infections; this is the more commonly utilized meaning of the word.

# MANY DIFFERENT TYPES OF BACTERIA MAKE US SICK

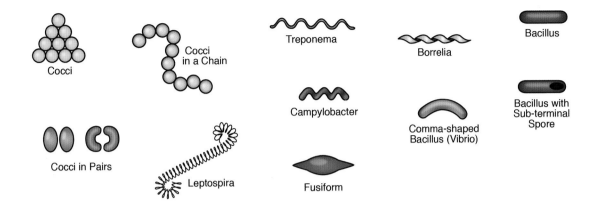

Bacteria that can make people sick are called **pathogenic**. **Only a small percentage of bacteria in the world actually cause disease in humans; even so, there are many different kinds of pathogenic bacteria.** Not all bacteria are shaped like the one on the previous page, but all bacteria are similarly complex in structure and are built up of similar components.

The ideal environment for each species of bacteria is also different: some prefer to attack us in our digestive area, causing vomiting and diarrhea, while others prefer to attack us in our ears, causing middle ear infections. Still others prefer to attack our skin, forming painful boils and skin infections. There are also a small group of bacteria which can thrive in multiple different environments.

When bacteria are suspected as the source of illness, identifying the specific type of bacteria involved is the first step in deciding which antibiotic to use for treatment.

# ANTIBIOTICS TARGET A SPECIFIC PART OF BACTERIA

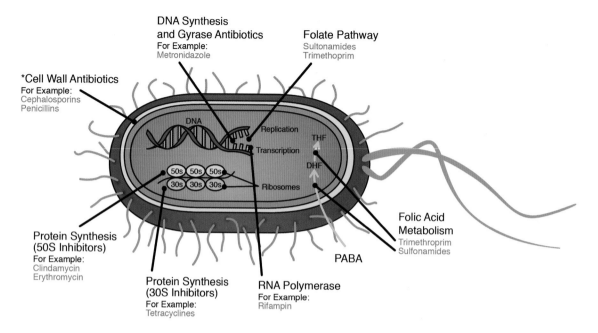

DNA Synthesis
and Gyrase Antibiotics
For Example:
Metronidazole

Folate Pathway
Sultonamides
Trimethoprim

*Cell Wall Antibiotics
For Example:
Cephalosporins
Penicillins

DNA

Replication

THF

Transcription

DHF

50s 50s 50s

30s 30s 30s

Ribosomes

Folic Acid
Metabolism
Trimethroprim
Sulfonamides

Protein Synthesis
(50S Inhibitors)
For Example:
Clindamycin
Erythromycin

PABA

Protein Synthesis
(30S Inhibitors)
For Example:
Tetracyclines

RNA Polymerase
For Example:
Rifampin

* Antibiotic classes are labeled in black. Individual antibiotics are labeled in red

In the majority of cases, when you have a bacterial infection, antibiotics should be administered to help fight the illness; while some bacterial illnesses *will* resolve without any medication, this should be carefully determined with the help of a doctor.

There are many different antibiotics available to treat bacteria. The picture above illustrates the many different classes of antibiotics, each targeting a different section of the bacteria. A single class of antibiotics may contain several different drugs, which all work very similarly.

**Picking an antibiotic for treatment is not "one-size-fits-all."** Each time a child is infected with a bacterial illness, the doctor must choose the best antibiotic to match the type of bacteria suspected. Often, an antibiotic class that works well against one group of bacteria will not work at all on a different group of bacteria.

In general, the most cost-effective antibiotic that best targets the germ suspected with the lowest potential for side effects should be utilized.

## YOUR BLOOD VESSELS ARE HIGHWAYS FOR GERMS

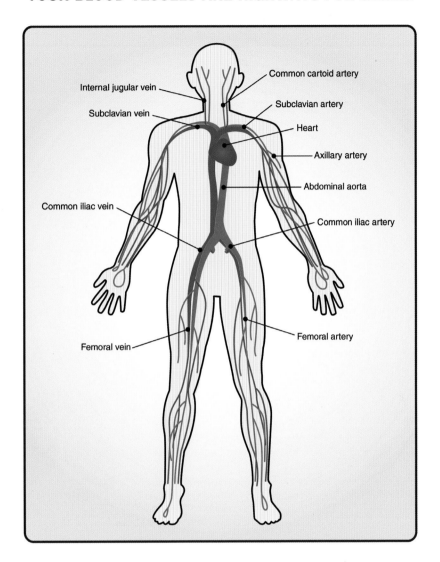

**Another very important factor in treating kids is ascertaining where the infection is located.** Your blood vessels provide a highway system for germs. A germ can enter the body from contact with animals, other people, infected surfaces, and even your own body. Once a germ enters your body, it can travel anywhere and infect virtually any organ in your body by following your bloodstream.

Knowing where in the body the infection is located can help determine what class of antibiotics should best be utilized, as certain antibiotics will better penetrate the specific organ that is infected.

# THE SAME GERM CAN PRESENT IN MULTIPLE WAYS

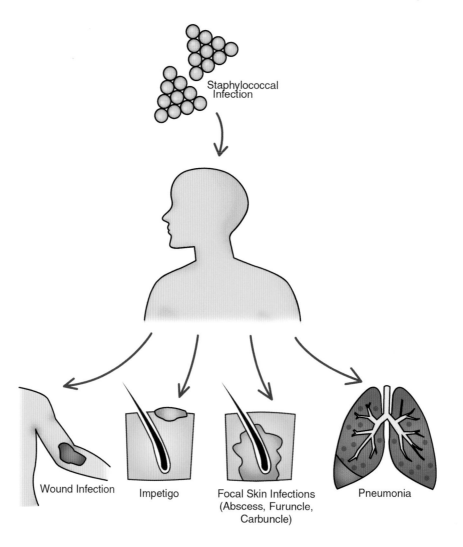

Staphylococcal Infection

Wound Infection

Impetigo

Focal Skin Infections (Abscess, Furuncle, Carbuncle)

Pneumonia

Germs can end up in different parts of the body, either transferred by external contact or by traveling through your blood vessels or other systems of your body.

**Depending on where the germ lands and seeds itself, the same germ can manifest as many different types of infections.**

For example, a staphylococcal bacterium can cause a pneumonia (infection of the lungs) if it seeds itself in the lungs. Alternatively, it can trigger several different types of skin infections (such as a wound infection, focal skin infection, or impetigo), depending on where it seeds itself in the skin. These are some of the more common examples in which the staphylococcal bacteria can infect an individual, but in reality almost any organ in the human body can be affected.

# WE HAVE MANY HEALTHY BACTERIA ON OUR BODY

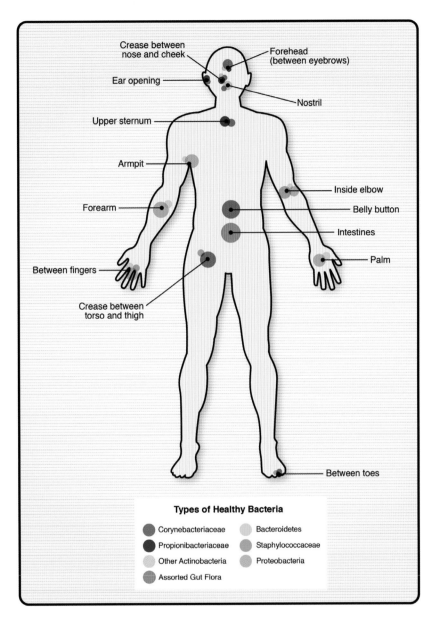

It is important to note that not all bacteria are bad. In fact, **our bodies are teeming with good bacteria that help keep us healthy.** Surprisingly, the number of overall bacterial cells (good and bad) in and on our bodies outnumbers our human cells tenfold.

Many of these good bacteria help maintain pH balance, crowd out bad bacteria, and assist with digestion and other bodily functions.

## ANTIBIOTICS DESTROY HEALTHY BACTERIA THAT AID IN DIGESTION

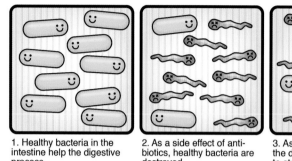

1. Healthy bacteria in the intestine help the digestive process

2. As a side effect of antibiotics, healthy bacteria are destroyed

3. As healthy bacteria return, the digestive process begins to stabilize

4. With time, the number of healthy bacteria returns back to the normal state

 Normal bacterium    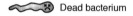 Dead bacterium

Our intestines, in particular, have many healthy bacteria that aid in our digestive process. This is why one of the side effects of taking antibiotics is diarrhea. **When you take antibiotics, in addition to killing off the bad bacteria that are causing the illness, you kill off healthy bacteria (for example, in the intestines).** After taking antibiotics, the digestive process becomes disrupted until the healthy bacteria are able to repopulate themselves in your intestines.

Another common side effect of taking antibiotics is developing a fungal skin infection. When the healthy bacteria occupying your skin are killed off, it makes it easier for a fungus to then invade the "vacant" skin cells.

Antibiotics can be lifesaving, but because of the potential side effects, it is important that they be used judiciously.

What to Know Before Seeing Your Pediatrician

## DISPLACEMENT OF COLONIZED BACTERIA CAN LEAD TO INFECTIONS

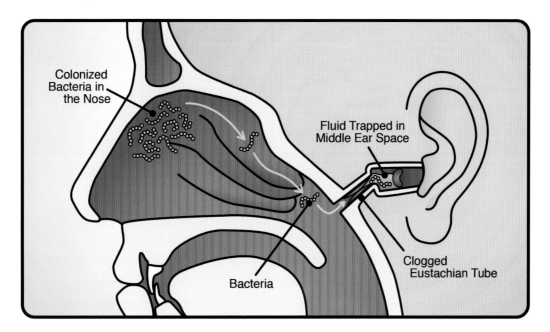

Some bacteria colonize themselves in certain parts of our bodies and live harmoniously with us, but they still have the potential to create trouble when they move to a different part of the body. For example, our nose harbors bacteria that are harmless—*if* they remain in place.

However, should the colonized bacteria from the nose become displaced and move to a different part of the body (such as the middle ear space), an infection can occur. **Bacterial infections often come from our own bodies when the germ "moves" from one part of the body to another.**

Another example of this happening is a skin infection. Many times, the germ that triggers the skin infection is already colonized somewhere else on our body. A cut or break in the skin allows the germ to burrow underneath the skin and fester, leading to a skin infection.

Parents often ask how their child acquired the germ that triggered their infection. Although we can acquire bacterial infections from contact with animals, other people, or infected surfaces, a lot of the time, the infection comes from the child's own body!

## OVERUSE OF ANTIBIOTICS CAN LEAD TO ANTIBIOTIC RESISTANCE

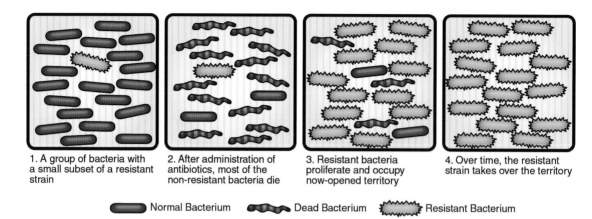

1. A group of bacteria with a small subset of a resistant strain

2. After administration of antibiotics, most of the non-resistant bacteria die

3. Resistant bacteria proliferate and occupy now-opened territory

4. Over time, the resistant strain takes over the territory

Normal Bacterium      Dead Bacterium      Resistant Bacterium

Another complication of antibiotics is that **resistant strains of bacteria can develop in your body over time.** When you take the same antibiotic over and over, natural selection goes to work on many of the bacteria that are colonized on your body, eventually selecting out only the bacteria that are resistant to that antibiotic.

Consider the colonized bacteria in your nose. Let's assume that 95 percent of the colonized bacteria can be killed with the antibiotic amoxicillin, while 5 percent of the colonized bacteria have resistance to amoxicillin, and as such, cannot be killed with amoxicillin (but can typically be killed with a stronger antibiotic*).

With every course of amoxicillin, the non-resistant strain of bacteria (the 95% which can be killed) will slowly decrease in population, while the resistant strain (the 5% which cannot be killed) will slowly increase in population, until your nose is completely colonized with only bacteria that are resistant to amoxicillin.

Should some of the colonized, antibiotic-resistant bacteria then "move" and create an infection in a different part of the body, the infection then becomes more difficult to treat because of its resistance to amoxicillin. Hence, a stronger antibiotic will be necessary, often carrying with it a larger potential for side effects.

---

*Some strains of antibiotic-resistant bacteria are only resistant to one or two antibiotics. Alarmingly, however, there are a growing number of bacteria that are resistant to all antibiotics and have no known treatment. While new antibiotics are in development, at present, this is a global healthcare issue that will require the cooperation of all nations in working toward the judicious use of antibiotics.

What to Know Before Seeing Your Pediatrician

The emergence of resistant strains of bacteria is why doctors must carefully choose the antibiotic that best targets the "bad" bacteria perpetrator, while minimizing the destruction of colonized bacteria that are not the cause of the acute infection being treated. In other words, when possible, it is always better to use a method with the least risk of collateral damage that can still get the job done.

## TAKE-HOME POINTS

★ Bacteria and viruses are different kinds of germs.

★ Antibiotics should only be used for bacteria, and do not work on viruses.

★ Antibiotics are not "one-size-fits-all."

★ Judicious use of antibiotics can minimize unwanted side effects and curb the rise of antibiotic-resistant bacteria.

In summary, although antibiotics are powerful weapons that can be lifesaving when used in the right situations, inappropriate use of them can lead to unwanted side effects and antibiotic resistance.

Because they target specific parts of bacteria, antibiotics will not work on viruses. The majority of infections seen in children are caused by viruses, which will typically get better with time, and which neither require nor respond to antibiotics.

# Chapter 2

# FEVER

THE PARENTAL fear that a doctor will probably encounter most often in the office is that of fever. **The textbook definition of fever is any temperature of 100.4°F or higher.** It is common for moms and dads to anxiously call the office anytime the thermometer reads 101°F or higher.

The good news is that the vast majority of fevers are not dangerous. Fevers can become dangerous when they reach **107.6°F** or higher, but this is rarely, if ever, seen in a pediatric office.

On the other hand, fevers spanning 100.4–106°F are seen several times a day in every pediatric office. Fevers in this range will not hurt the brain. Many moms and dads have heard of a fever triggering seizures, and although this can be alarming to the parent, the good news is that simple **febrile seizures** (a seizure associated with a fever) are not dangerous, and typically have no lasting effects; this is in contrast to other types of seizures, which can be more concerning.

Fevers are a natural and healthy response of the immune system. A solid understanding of what a fever is will help parents not to panic the next time their child gets sick, and may even save them a visit to the doctor.

## HOW FEVER IS TRIGGERED

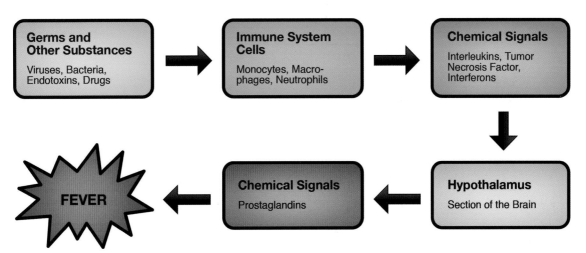

The pathway to fever is an intentional series of chemical signals orchestrated by the brain. Germs (or other foreign substances) entering the body are the typical source of fever. **Fever is purposefully created by the body to help our immune system fight a germ more efficiently.** In other words, fevers are **beneficial in fighting off germs**.

If this is true, then should a fever-reducer be used at all?

Great question!

If a child is comfortable and able to drink liquids in order to stay hydrated, it is probably better not to use any type of medication to keep the fever down.

However, an uncomfortable child may refuse liquids, which can lead to dehydration; as such, although the fever is being helpful in fighting off germs, the child who is refusing liquids should be treated with a fever-reducer, as it is more important to keep the child well hydrated.

It is also perfectly reasonable to use fever-reducers purely for the comfort of a child. Although there is a small trade-off in reducing the efficiency of the child's immune system, a comfortable night's rest can also go a long way in fighting off a germ.

Lukewarm baths and cool cloths on foreheads can also help to comfort a child, but in general, outside of fever-reducing medications, other interventions do not work well in bringing down the core temperature of the body.

Some parents debate whether to bundle up or strip down a feverish child. It is probably best to do whatever feels most comfortable for the child at that particular time. In the course of a single illness, there may be moments when an extra blanket feels more comfortable, and times when prancing around in one's underwear feels the best.

## FEVER IS A CONTROLLED BURN

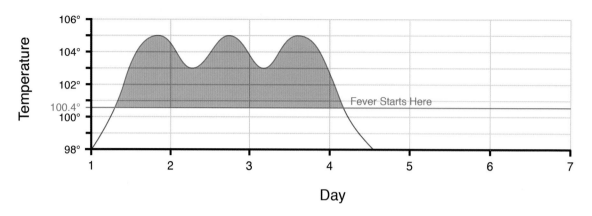

One of the reasons that parents are fearful of fever is because they fail to realize that **a fever is a controlled burn.** The body has a feedback loop with the brain to ensure that the fever does not become "too hot." Parents sometimes become overly vigilant about bringing a fever down and, as a result, do more harm than good by overusing fever-reducers (and incurring possible side effects).

Even without any intervention (including fever-reducing medications), fevers will stay in a specific range and will not spiral out of control. The fever will eventually break as the infection is defeated, and the body temperature will return to normal.

But, as we have discussed, because fever can make a child uncomfortable, it is perfectly reasonable to make use of fever-reducing medications and other techniques (such as baths) to help make a child feel better. However, intervention is not necessary to control the fever; the body will do that on its own.

**A good motto for using fever-reducing medications is, "Treat the child, not the fever."** In other words, a child who is playful but has a 103°F fever does not necessarily need any medication. Conversely, a child who is uncomfortable, but who only has a 101°F fever would benefit from medication (for comfort purposes).

## CONTROLLING THE FEVER WILL NOT REDUCE
## THE LIKELIHOOD OF A FEBRILE SEIZURE

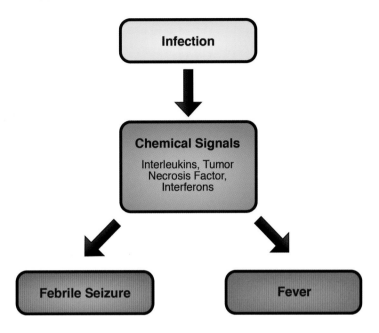

One of the reasons many parents are afraid of fevers is because they have all heard of a child who has experienced a febrile seizure. A child experiencing a febrile seizure will be unconscious and appear to have their eyes rolling backward. Initially, their entire body will be stiff, but eventually this will progress to twitching and shaking. **While a febrile seizure appears dangerous, *simple febrile seizures are benign, and leave no long-term damage.*** They are also quite common; nearly 5 percent of children will have a febrile seizure at least once in their lifetime, and many will have more than one.

Once their child *has* had a febrile seizure, parents will aggressively attempt to control all future fevers. However, it is likely that febrile seizures are not actually triggered by the fevers themselves, but are rather triggered by the same chemical signal pathway that led to the fever; thus, even if you control the fever, the chemical signals can still trigger the seizure. **Studies have shown that aggressive management of fever will not prevent a febrile seizure.**

Febrile seizures should be evaluated by a doctor but often do not require emergency care. When a febrile seizure occurs, place the child on their side and on the ground away from harmful objects. Do not try to place anything in their mouth, as there is no risk of swallowing the tongue. Time the seizure. If it lasts 5 minutes or longer, call 911. Most febrile seizures will last 1–2 minutes—although it will feel much longer! Once the seizure has ended, call a doctor for further instructions.

A visit to the emergency room for a febrile seizure is generally unnecessary, unless other risk factors are present. It is unclear why some children are prone to febrile seizures. The good news is that even for children who are prone to febrile seizures, not every fever will trigger a seizure and most will outgrow them by 5 years of age.

It is important to note that a **simple febrile seizure** is different from a **complex febrile seizure**. A complex febrile seizure is defined as multiple febrile seizures in a 24-hour period, or a febrile seizure that lasts longer than 15 minutes. Additionally, a **focal febrile seizure** is also considered a complex febrile seizure, and is more concerning than a **generalized seizure**. A focal seizure is when a discrete part of the body is twitching by itself, as opposed to a generalized seizure where the entire body twitches and shakes. **All complex febrile seizures should receive immediate medical attention.**

# FEVER DECISION TREE

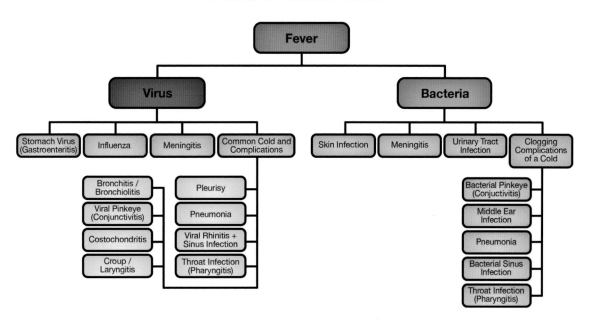

If doctors are not concerned about the fever itself, then what is going through their head when examining a child with a fever? In general, **the doctor is trying to figure out what kind of infection is triggering the fever.** While the doctor is asking questions and examining a child, they are running through a checklist of possible infections and mentally eliminating those that don't fit (as shown above).

If the fever is triggered by a **common virus**, there is unlikely to be any harm from the infection itself, unless a major organ (such as the brain, heart, lungs, or liver) is being attacked. The vast majority of viral infections will resolve on their own without any intervention, meaning there is little to be done.

If the fever is triggered by **bacteria**, however, there is greater cause for concern. Most bacterial illnesses require antibiotics. If the infection is left untreated, it can oftentimes worsen and lead to harm. Prompt treatment is imperative, especially if bacteria are invading a major organ (such as the brain, heart, lungs, or kidneys).

With common illnesses, distinguishing between a bacterial and viral infection will be easy enough for an experienced parent to discern. However, there will be times that a doctor's expertise and a physical exam will be needed to help with the determination. Judicious use of tests (such as a strep throat swab or urine/blood tests) may also be helpful; however, an experienced doctor will often not need tests to confirm the diagnosis.

## INFANT SICKNESS GAUGE

|  | Energy | Interaction | Appetite |
|---|---|---|---|
| **Strong** | Normal activites; mobile around the home | Coos, laughs, and smiles | Normal |
| **Moderate** | Sits and holds up head per normal ability | Intermittent smiling with good eye contact | Drinks formula/breast milk freely but little interest in solid food |
| **Weak** | Lays in bed with minimal activity | Minimal smiling and little eye contact | Must be encouraged to drink anything |

## CHILD SICKNESS GAUGE

|  | Energy | Interaction | Appetite |
|---|---|---|---|
| **Strong** | Normal activities; walks around the house | Talks freely | Normal |
| **Moderate** | Interested in TV; can sit comfortably | Minimal talking but normal amount of eye contact | Drinks freely but little interest in solid food |
| **Weak** | Lies in bed with minimal activity | Little talking and little eye contact | Must be encouraged to drink or eat anything |

What to Know Before Seeing Your Pediatrician

# GAUGING THE SERIOUSNESS OF AN ILLNESS

So, does *every* fever need to be seen by the doctor? NO! Most fevers do *not* need an evaluation by the doctor. As parents become more experienced with their child's illnesses, they will be able to determine whether a visit to the doctor is necessary, or if monitoring the child at home will suffice.

**More important than the actual measurement of the fever is the activity level of the child.** Put simply, a child with a serious infection will not play! Rather, a child with a serious infection will get worse from day to day. A child with a serious infection will perk up minimally with a fever-reducer (it may take 30–60 minutes for the medication to kick in).

These charts can help to gauge the activity level of a child. The more active they are, the more they talk, and the more they eat—the less you have to worry. The less active they are, the less they talk, and the less they eat—the *more* you have to worry.

Again, **it is not necessary to treat a fever.** However, fever-reducers are helpful in making the child more comfortable and in gauging how sick a child truly is. If a child perks up after taking a fever-reducer, there is little to be worried about. If a child does not perk up after taking a fever-reducer, while it does not necessarily indicate the presence of a serious infection, parents should closely monitor the child and call or visit the doctor to touch base.

**Please note that for any infant 3 months of age or younger, any fever of 100.4°F or higher should be reported to the doctor as soon as possible.** Young infants give fewer clues that indicate how sick they truly are. Additionally, because they have an immature immune system and have not yet received all their vaccinations, it is imperative to thoroughly assess newborn babies to rule out any serious source of infection. Even in newborns, it is not the height of the fever that is worrisome—it is the possibility that the fever represents a serious infection that most concerns the doctor.

## TAKING THE RECTAL TEMPERATURE OF AN INFANT

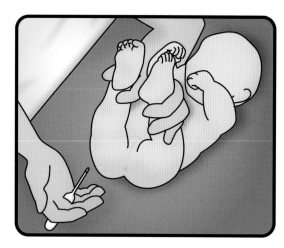 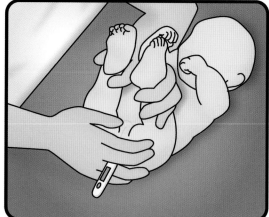

For babies younger than 3 months of age, the best place to check the temperature is in the rectum (any thermometer designed for taking rectal temperatures is appropriate). For babies older than 3 months, other methods are reasonable. Often, when parents measure the baby's temperature somewhere other than the rectum, they feel they should add or subtract a degree. **When measuring a temperature, it is better not to add or subtract a degree, but to report it as shown by the thermometer.**

Noting when the temperature was taken, where the temperature was measured, and when the last time a fever-reducing medication was administered can also be useful information. A simple chart documenting these items can be very helpful.

**In children 1 year and older, because activity level is a better gauge for how sick a child truly is, precise temperature measurements are not as important.** Any modality of thermometers is reasonable, and vigilant temperature checking is generally not needed.

What to Know Before Seeing Your Pediatrician

# HOW TO TAKE A RECTAL TEMPERATURE

1. Lubricate the tip of the thermometer with a lubricating jelly.

2. Lay the baby down (facing up) on a firm flat surface, such as a changing table.

3. Grab the baby's legs securely with one hand.

4. Place the thermometer firmly between the second and third fingers of the free hand.

5. Insert the lubricated thermometer through the anal opening, about ½–1 inch (about 1.25–2.5 centimeters) into the rectum. Stop at less than ½ inch (about 1.25 centimeters) if you feel any resistance.

6. Steady the thermometer between your second and third fingers as you cup your hand against your baby's bottom. Soothe your baby and speak to them quietly as you hold the thermometer in place.

7. Wait until you hear the appropriate number of beeps or any other signal indicating that the temperature is ready to be read. Read and record the number on the screen, noting the time of day that the reading was taken.

## ALTERNATING FEVER MEDICATIONS

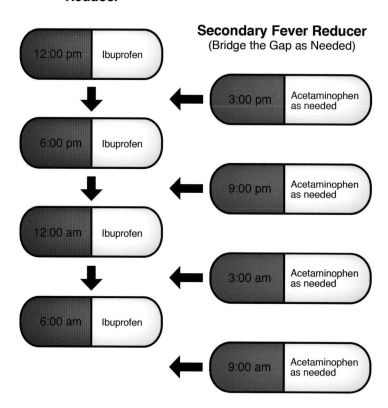

**Primary Fever Reducer**

**Secondary Fever Reducer**
(Bridge the Gap as Needed)

12:00 pm — Ibuprofen

3:00 pm — Acetaminophen as needed

6:00 pm — Ibuprofen

9:00 pm — Acetaminophen as needed

12:00 am — Ibuprofen

3:00 am — Acetaminophen as needed

6:00 am — Ibuprofen

9:00 am — Acetaminophen as needed

As previously mentioned, fever-reducing medication should be used for the purpose of keeping a child comfortable. For children, the two most commonly used fever-reducers are ibuprofen (Motrin and Advil are examples) and acetaminophen (Tylenol). Ibuprofen and acetaminophen work similarly; however, ibuprofen is mainly metabolized by the kidneys, and acetaminophen is metabolized by the liver. Aspirin (which is different from ibuprofen and acetaminophen) should never be given to children except in rare circumstances when instructed by a doctor.

A good approach with fever-reducers is to use only one medication and use it no more than every six hours. If the child appears uncomfortable at the three- to four-hour mark between doses, a second alternative fever-reducer can be used, as needed, to bridge the gap.

For example, a mother could use ibuprofen at 12 pm, 6 pm, 12 am, 6 am and so forth. At 3 pm or 9 pm, if needed, she can use acetaminophen to bridge the gap.

In general, it is best to stick to just one medication. Alternating medications frequently can lead to confusion: There may be miscommunication between parents or forgetfulness, which can result in giving the same medication every three hours instead of every six, leading to accidental overdosing. Overuse of acetaminophen can lead to liver damage, and overuse of ibuprofen can lead to kidney (and in rare cases, liver) damage. A written record of what medication was given at what time can help prevent errors.

**Studies show that using one medication works just as well as two in terms of keeping a child comfortable—so err on the side of using just one!** Anecdotally, ibuprofen seems to work better than acetaminophen.

## TAKE-HOME POINTS

★ Fevers under 107.6°F are not dangerous; in fact, fever is actually *beneficial*.

★ Fever is a controlled burn.

★ Treat the child for comfort, not for the fever.

★ Simple febrile seizures are not dangerous.

★ The source of the fever is more important than the fever itself.

★ Activity is a better gauge of sickness than the actual number of the fever.

★ Alternating different fever-reducers is acceptable, but using a single medicine is preferable.

Fever is a controlled burn that the body will regulate; however, fever-reducers can be used to keep a child comfortable until the germ is defeated. Any child who appears to be getting worse over time should be evaluated by a doctor.

Understanding the role of fever in the body can help reduce parental anxiety and prevent the possible side effects from overuse of fever-reducing medications.

Most children will experience fevers throughout the course of their childhood. In and of itself, fever is not dangerous. The most important part of evaluating a fever is to identify the source of the fever. Gauging a child's energy, interactions, and appetite can help determine the seriousness of the illness.

# Chapter 3

# VACCINES

WITHOUT A doubt, vaccines and vaccination represent the greatest medical advancement in recent history. The number of lives saved and people kept healthy as a result of vaccines is astounding.

In the United States, prior to immunizations, each year approximately 500 people died of measles, 200,000 cases of whooping cough were reported, and 20,000 people became paralyzed from polio.

Conversely, in the United States in 2011, there were no deaths from measles, less than 20,000 cases of whooping cough reported, and zero cases of paralysis from polio. And these are just a few of the diseases for which vaccines have improved the overall health and well-being of society.

Unfortunately, vaccines are a victim of their own success. Today, more and more parents are refusing vaccines for themselves and their children, never having witnessed the horrific effects of measles, polio, diphtheria, and other diseases. Much of the fear of vaccines is predicated on misinformation that is circulated by websites maintained by individuals with few medical credentials.

This is not to say that there are *no* risks with vaccines. The Centers for Disease Control and Prevention (CDC) has a webpage dedicated to outlining the various risks with each vaccine ranging from serious allergic reactions to the most common side effect, redness and irritation at the injection site.

Vaccines are neither foolproof nor 100 percent safe; but like many aspects of medicine (or life, for that matter), the risk must be weighed against the benefit. In the case of vaccines, any doctor who practices evidence-based medicine will attest to what the scientific literature has clearly demonstrated: The benefits of vaccines overwhelmingly outweigh the risks.

# THE SUCCESS OF THE POLIOVIRUS VACCINE
# PROVES THE POWER OF IMMUNIZATIONS

### Progress in Polio Eradication
### Global Wild Poliovirus Cases, 1988-2006

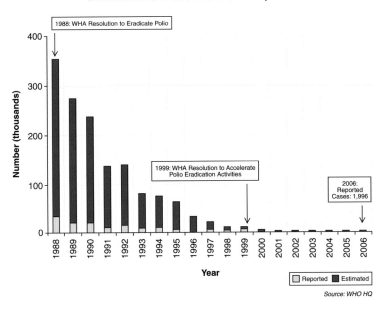

Source: WHO HQ

After smallpox (which has been eradicated for over 30 years), the polio vaccine best demonstrates the far-reaching health effects of a successful vaccine. The poliovirus vaccine was first widely used in industrial countries in the 1950s. Since then, global eradication of the poliovirus is nearly within reach, and represents one of the greatest success stories regarding vaccines.

In the United States, the number of paralytic poliomyelitis cases declined from more than 20,000 cases in 1952 to fewer than 100 cases in the mid-1960s. The last documented indigenous case of wild poliovirus in the Unites States was in 1979!

In 1988, the World Health Assembly set out to globally eradicate the poliovirus by the year 2000. **Although this goal was not met, it seems it is only a matter of time before poliovirus joins smallpox on the list of eradicated and extinct viruses.**

# THE MEASLES VACCINE IS ANOTHER SUCCESS STORY OF IMMUNIZATIONS

### Measles - United States, 1950-2004

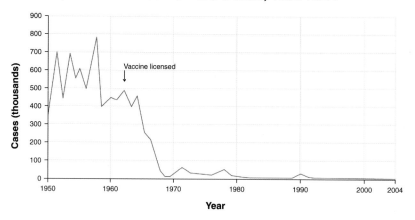

*Epidemiology and Prevention of Vaccine - Preventable Diseases January 2006*

Another great example of the prowess of immunizations is the measles vaccine. This graph clearly demonstrates the power of the measles vaccine in the United States since its introduction in 1963. However, measles is still fairly prevalent throughout the world, and has lately been making a small comeback in certain areas due to unsubstantiated fears about the vaccine.

In 1998, Andrew Wakefield made a fraudulent claim linking the measles, mumps, and rubella vaccine (MMR) with autism. Allegedly, Dr. Wakefield falsified data for use in a lawsuit against vaccine producers. It was later discovered that Dr. Wakefield had a serious conflict of interest in his research—he was planning to launch a business venture based around an autism diagnostic kit, from which he would have profited by discrediting the MMR immunization.

The fraudulent paper fueled a sharp decrease in immunization rates, which has subsequently led to repeated outbreaks of measles in pockets throughout the world. In the aftermath, Wakefield lost his medical license, the medical journal retracted the original research paper, and multiple studies have discredited his findings.

Unfortunately, vaccine fear-mongering is still a current issue, with new websites being assisted by shoddy science, filling the void left behind by Wakefield's report. **Vaccines are not without their risk; however, the risk-to-benefit ratio overwhelmingly favors receiving all current immunizations recommended by the CDC.**

Polio and measles are just two examples of how successful vaccines have been in improving the overall health of society. Parents can learn about the full list of recommended vaccines and how these immunizations can protect their children at www.cdc.gov.

# HOW VACCINES WORK

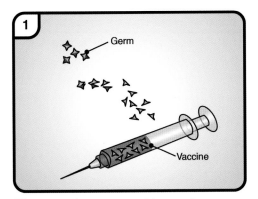

The germ is processed to create a vaccine

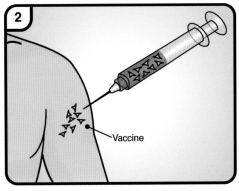

A vaccine is injected into the body

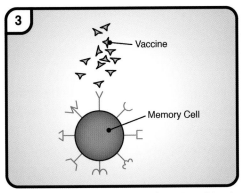

The vaccine particle attaches to a blank memory cell

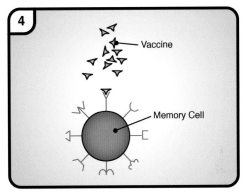

The vaccine particle triggers the memory cell to create a certain shape of antibodies

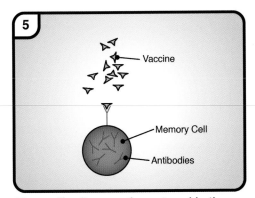

The antibodies are then stored in the memory cell until they are needed

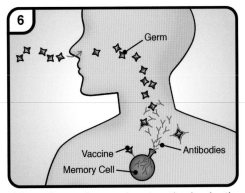

When the real germ invates the body, the memory cell releases the antibodies to combat the infection

**Vaccines work by triggering the natural immune system of the body.** A vaccine is usually a piece of the actual germ that causes disease; alternatively, it can be a weakened version of the germ itself.

The goal is to use the vaccine particle to "trick" the immune system into making and storing memory cells. These cells will then be ready to fight the actual germ, should it be encountered in the future. Memory cells are a component of your immune system, and are essentially factories for weapons called antibodies. Antibodies are powerful weapons that attach to germs as soon as they are detected in the body. Once an antibody attaches to a germ, it triggers the immune system to destroy and dispose of the germ. The more memory cells a body has stored and ready to fight a germ, the sooner the body will get rid of the real germ if and when it invades.

Another way to think about immunizations is that they are training for your immune system. Imagine an army, belonging to any country in the world. Getting sick from a germ is analogous to this country being invaded by another country's armed forces. If the defending army has never been trained against their enemy's tactics, the chances of winning the battle are small, especially if the invading enemy deploys powerful weapons. But, if the defense has gone through rigorous training, **simulating actual battlefield conditions**, they will be far better prepared and much more likely to be victorious. Importantly, it will also minimize the collateral damage to their home country.

In an ideal world, a single dose of any vaccine would be all the training the immune system would require to provide lifelong protection against the targeted germ. **The unfortunate reality is that most vaccines require several booster shots of the same vaccine to build up a sufficient amount of memory cells to properly fight future infections.** Some vaccines only need a single lifetime booster (two immunizations total), while other vaccines require a booster immunization every 10 years, for life.

## THE IMMUNE SYSTEM IS GOOD AT MULTI-TASKING

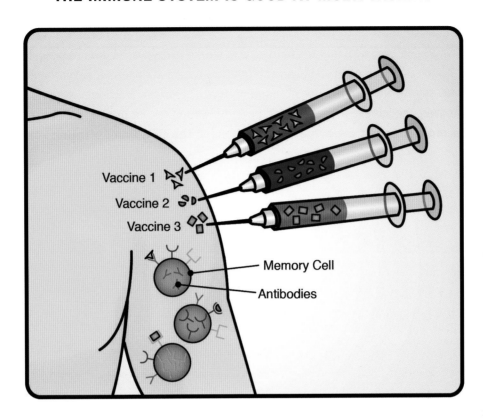

As science improves, we are discovering more and more vaccines to protect our bodies against deadly diseases. The standard immunization schedule is constantly expanding to include new vaccines, providing a healthier and better future for the next generation. In order to maximize protection against a plethora of germs, many of the early check-ups for children now provide multiple vaccines at each visit.

The good news is that **the immune system is superb at multi-tasking.** For example, consider how many germs and foreign invaders the body encounters on a daily basis as a child travels from home, to school, to the outdoors, and back home again. The immune system must encounter, filter, and fight hundreds of different invaders each day to keep the body healthy. Similarly, our immune system can easily handle multiple vaccines at one time in a safe and efficient manner—in reality, it is no different from a regular day's work for your immune system.

One false concern (which has become a mainstream opinion) is that multiple vaccines at one visit can potentially be harmful, and that it is safer to break up the vaccine schedule so that only one or two vaccines are administered per visit. If done methodically, this is a reasonable (but not beneficial) alternative to the standard schedule. However, there are risks involved in employing an alternative vaccine schedule, and it is generally not recommended.

Firstly, it delays protection by postponing some vaccines. Secondly, it creates more visits to the doctor's office. Research shows that the sum total of stress to children is greater when they have to return more frequently for one or two shots at a time, as opposed to getting several immunizations in fewer visits. Thirdly, there is greater potential for clerical error when a known routine is traded for an alternative schedule.

**Optimal protection is best achieved by following the CDC immunization schedule.**

# WHY AN ANNUAL FLU VACCINE IS NEEDED

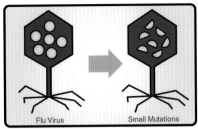

Antigenic Drift

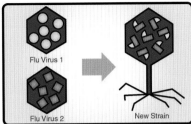

Antigenic Shift

Although many vaccines require booster immunizations, the only one that currently requires an **annual booster** is the flu (influenza) vaccine. Unlike other germs, which tend to look the same year after year, the flu virus is the great chameleon, changing its appearance on a regular basis.

**The flu virus uses two methods to change its shape: antigenic drift and antigenic shift.** Using these two methods, it has the ability to constantly reinvent itself, changing the very proteins against which we vaccinate.

Every spring, the World Health Organization valiantly attempts to predict what flu viruses will look like in the upcoming winter season (there is often more than one strain circulating). It selects 3–4 different strains of the flu virus to be targeted by the vaccine, with some being similar to the years prior, and others being tweaked to reflect ongoing surveillance data. It is a difficult task, to say the least.

The eventual goal is to create a flu vaccine that attacks a protein on the virus that does not change shape from year to year—but thus far, this goal continues to elude scientists.

Understandably, families are wary of receiving a flu vaccine year after year. However, it is important not to underestimate the annual threat of the flu virus. Each year, there are up to 36,000 flu-related deaths in the United States alone, with approximately 100 of them occurring in children younger than 5 years of age. The best protection is to maintain vigilance by receiving the annual flu vaccine.

In addition to safeguarding against the flu, an added benefit of the flu vaccine is that it confers a protective effect against middle ear infections, sinus infections, and pneumonia. Anecdotally, many people have come down with the common cold soon after receiving a flu vaccine, and mistakenly blame the vaccine for making them sick. Although it is not uncommon to feel pain at the injection site and some fatigue for one or two days following the immunization, the vaccine itself cannot actually make you sick.

The injectable vaccine is made up of flu particles or an inactivated (killed) virus; thus, it is impossible to become ill from the injection. The nasal flu vaccine is a weakened version of a live flu virus; however, the weakened virus is cold-adapted, meaning the virus is designed to only reside long enough in the nose (where temperatures are cooler) to trigger a proper immune response. It cannot infect the lungs, or other areas where the temperature is warmer; thus, it is also not possible to become ill from the nasal vaccine.

# HERD IMMUNITY HELPS PROTECT THE UNVACCINATED BABY

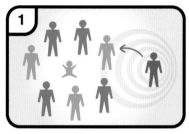 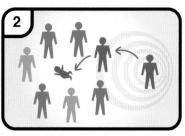 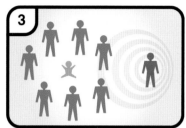

If only SOME get vaccinated, the germ spreads and infects the infant

If ALL get vaccinated, the germ is contained and the infant is safe

Healthy, non-vaccinated    Healthy, vaccinated    Non-vaccinated, sick, contagious

The vaccine schedule starts at birth, when the newborn receives the first Hepatitis B vaccine. The baby will then receive multiple immunizations at 2, 4, and 6 months. In the first few months of life (until the vaccines produce protective immunity), the infant is vulnerable to many diseases. Furthermore, certain vaccines (particularly the live virus vaccines and the flu vaccine) cannot be given until the child is older, which delays protection against these illnesses as well.

Thus, it is important in the first few months of life to promote herd immunity until all the important vaccines are given. **Herd immunity means that all caretakers who interact regularly with the baby have received vaccines against diseases to which the baby is susceptible, protecting the infant from being exposed to those specific germs.**

In the United States, the Tdap booster (for whooping cough protection) and the flu vaccine are probably the most important vaccines to receive for herd immunization. Other vaccines to consider are Hepatitis A, MMR (Measles/Mumps/Rubella), and Chicken Pox (Varicella). The better immunized a family is, the less risk there is to the infant until they acquire their own protection through the CDC immunization schedule.

Herd immunity is absolutely important for infants, but it is equally vital for individuals in our society with weakened immune systems, whether it be from cancer treatment, a hereditary condition, or an infection. The ideal way for individuals with weak immune systems to be protected is for those of us with normal immune systems to stay vigilant in receiving our vaccines.

# TAKE-HOME POINTS

★ The benefits of vaccines clearly outweigh the risks.

★ Immune systems can multitask and handle multiple vaccines at one time.

★ Optimal protection is best achieved by following the CDC immunization schedule.

★ The changing nature of the flu virus necessitates an annual flu shot.

★ Herd immunity is important for babies and those who cannot receive vaccines.

When immunization rates reach high levels, disease rates drop and the dangerous outcomes of these diseases fade from the public memory. While this is a public health success, it unfortunately makes it easier for parents to become lax about following the recommended vaccine schedule.

Over time, immunization rates drop, leaving more and more people in society unprotected, thereby increasing risk for outbreaks. Eventually, diseases that were once well under control will start to break out in small epidemics.

Those with immune systems that are not robust, including young babies, rely upon herd immunity to stay free of disease. In order to protect those members of society who cannot receive immunizations, it is imperative for those of us who *can* to stay vigilant.

Even from the individual's own health perspective, becoming fully immunized is the healthiest and safest decision that an individual can make for oneself. Ultimately, risks must always be weighed against benefits, and in terms of immunizations, research has shown more clearly than ever that the best thing for the individual—and society as a whole—is to get protected by getting vaccinated.

What to Know Before Seeing Your Pediatrician

# Chapter 4

# THE COMMON COLD

ONE OF the most vexing aspects of pediatrics is dealing with the common cold. Everyone gets it, everyone suffers from it, and everyone hates it, yet there is not much that modern medicine has to offer in terms of treatment.

The common cold leads to coughing, sneezing, runny nose, sore throat, congestion, and fever. There are countless drugstore medications and homemade remedies that people take to combat a cold. Unfortunately, little evidence supports their effectiveness. Most children will get 6–8 colds (or more) per year; thankfully, all of them will go away with time and require little intervention.

It is important to understand the common cold thoroughly, however, because it is a gateway infection that can lead to a host of other complications commonly seen in pediatrics. There are two categories into which all complications of the common cold fit: **inflammatory complications** and **clogging complications**.

Inflammatory complications (see page 51) of the cold occur when the invading virus inflames any part of the respiratory tract, starting from the mouth all the way down to the alveoli (air sacs) of the lung. This can lead to nasal inflammation (rhinitis), a viral sinus infection, a viral throat infection, croup, laryngitis, bronchitis, bronchiolitis, a viral pneumonia, or a viral pinkeye (conjunctivitis). Although these complications cannot be cured by antibiotics, things can be done to help monitor, comfort, and sometimes treat the child.

Clogging complications (see Chapters 5 and 6) occur when colds create mucus and congestion. This can lead to blockage of various drainage pipes in the body, creating stagnant fluid and allowing bacteria to fester and multiply. This can lead to an ear infection, a bacterial sinus infection, a bacterial pneumonia, or a bacterial pinkeye. Clogging-induced infections are initially triggered by a viral cold, but subsequently will involve bacteria and thus often require antibiotics; whereas when dealing with just the common cold, which is caused by a virus, antibiotics are neither needed nor helpful.

Understanding how colds typically improve and go away on their own, or else evolve into complications, can help a parent distinguish when a child can stay at home and duke it out, versus when a child needs to be evaluated by a doctor for possible intervention.

# MANY DIFFERENT COLD VIRUSES MAKE US SICK

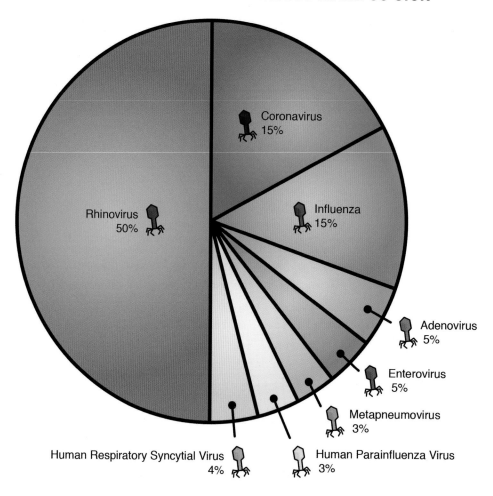

Unlike some viruses, such as the chicken pox, which is typically contracted only once, the common cold can be caught over and over and over (and over and over). **There are more than 200 different types of cold viruses that can make you sick.**

Even if you successfully suffer through and fight off one cold, there are a slew of other viruses ready to attack you as soon as you get better—often in succession, with no break in between. As previously stated, most kids will get 6–8 colds per year; for those who attend a daycare-type setting, the number can be even higher, ranging between 8 and 12 colds per year (or more).

As you get older, and your body has encountered and successfully combated many of the different cold viruses, your immune system will become wiser and more experienced. Unfortunately for children, this wisdom and experience can only come by going through the numerous battles. It may take several years before the frequency of yearly colds begins to mitigate.

## COLDS ARE MORE PREVALENT DURING THE WINTERTIME

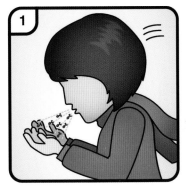 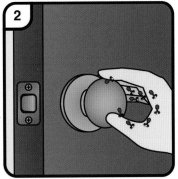 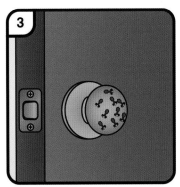

Cold viruses tend to travel and spread more easily when the humidity is low, which is most common during the wintertime. Viruses can be passed via surfaces such as door handles, keyboards, and shopping carts. People also tend to congregate indoors more frequently during the wintertime, thus increasing the transfer rate of viruses. For this reason, the bulk of colds kids will catch happen during the winter months.

The cold temperature itself does not make you sick. **Cold weather leads to decreased humidity and indoor crowding, which subsequently increases the transfer of cold viruses.** If no cold viruses are passed from person to person, regardless of how cold it is, you will not become sick.

That being said, although the cold weather by itself cannot make you sick, new research suggests that the cold weather may make it easier for cold viruses to replicate within your body. The cold weather may also weaken your immune defenses, making it easier for the cold virus to invade your body.

So, perhaps there *is* some truth to grandma telling you to bundle up during the wintertime so that you won't get sick! Remember, though: No matter how cold it is outside, it is the presence of the cold virus that precipitates the illness, not the cold weather itself.

# THE COLD VIRUS IS SPREAD BY TOUCH, SNEEZES, AND COUGH

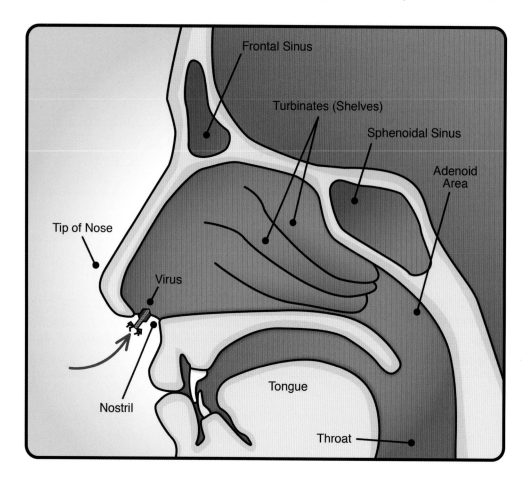

The cold virus is virtually everywhere during the fall and winter. Even the most diligent hand-washing family will still catch several colds every winter. It is an unavoidable part of life.

The typical cold virus is picked up when your hand touches a surface that was previously infected by another person. The cold virus is now on your hand, and subsequent contact with your nose, mouth, or eyes will give the virus an entryway into your body.

Cold viruses can also attack through the air. When someone with a cold sneezes or coughs, the expelled saliva carries cold viruses through the air, with the potential to infect surrounding people.

**The high prevalence of the cold virus makes it nearly impossible to avoid the common cold during the wintertime.** The good news is that colds are not dangerous (unless complications ensue), and the act of your immune system fighting off a cold is actually healthy and beneficial for the body.

Of course, practicing good hygiene habits, while not a perfect defense, can still reduce the overall number of colds and other germs that a family catches throughout the year. A good habit to teach your kids is to wash their hands regularly for the duration of the "Happy Birthday" song, and to dry them thoroughly afterward. Children should also be taught to sneeze into their elbows rather than their hands, to reduce the transmission of germs to others.

# HOW THE COLD VIRUS DAMAGES THE INNER SKIN CELLS

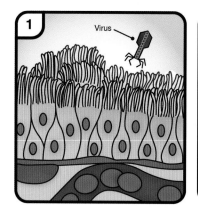
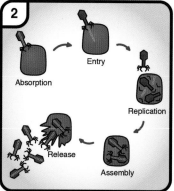
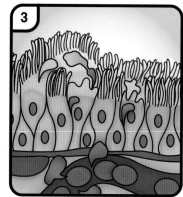

Once the cold virus infiltrates your body through your nose, mouth, or eyes, it begins its work of reproducing itself by taking over your inner skin cells. Through a constant process of infiltrating and replicating, the cold virus destroys many of the body's cells in the area of infection.

When you fall down and skin your knee, no amount of medications will accelerate the healing process of the knee's skin—it takes time for the new skin cells to grow back! In the same way, **when a cold virus destroys the inner skin cells in your nose, throat, or eyes, no amount of medication is going to accelerate the healing process.** Healing will happen with time, but there will be mucus and irritation until the skin is restored.

There are many cough and cold medications that claim to help relieve the congestion and cough associated with the common cold. Decongestants purportedly reduce nasal congestion by shrinking the blood vessels in your nose, so that less mucus is produced, while cough medications are supposed to act on the cough center in our brain to depress the cough reflex.

**Neither group of medications helps the healing process, nor have they been proven to work in children.** Furthermore, many of these medications are actually known to trigger dangerous side effects. For these reasons, cough and cold medications should *never* be given to children.

## POOR DRAINAGE OF MUCUS MAKES COUGH WORSE AT NIGHT

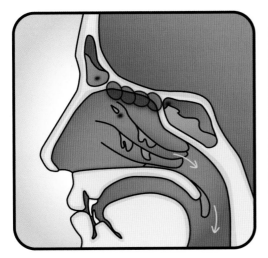 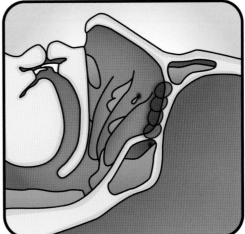

Because we are vertical during the day, mucus drains down the throat and coughing is kept at a minimum. **However, at night when we are lying down, mucus pools in the back of the throat, making it hard to breathe and triggering nighttime coughing.** The typical pattern parents observe are periods of sleeping interrupted by bouts of heavy coughing throughout the night.

What is happening is that, after lying down, the back of the throat slowly fills up with mucus, like a swimming pool being filled with water. Once the pool of mucus reaches a certain threshold point, the body triggers a bout of coughing to help protect the airway from being inundated with fluids, after which the cycle repeats itself all over again.

Remember, medications do *not* help control the mucus and are not safe for children—particularly those younger than the age of 6 years. Some safe things can be done for comfort, but it is important to bear in mind that ultimately, time is the great healer.

1. Suction the nose as often as the child will tolerate to help keep mucus to a minimum. Electronic devices and those powered by the sucking power of a parent's mouth can be particularly helpful. Nasal saline drops can be used to help break up the mucus for easier suctioning.

2. Keep children upright or have them sleep at an angle at night to help gravity move the mucus downward. For older children, this can be done by using an extra pillow or two. Discuss some safe options for your baby with your doctor.

3. A humidifier at night may help mask the tickling feeling in the back of the throat and may also keep the mucus from becoming too thick.

4. For children *over* 1 year of age, 1–2 teaspoons of honey can be given as often as needed and may also help mask the tickling feeling in the back of the throat. **(Do not give honey to children younger than 1 year of age because of the risk of botulism.)**

5. Make sure you keep your child well hydrated with plenty of fluids. A bowl of grandma's chicken noodle soup never hurts, and the steam may even help to break up the mucus.

# THE COMMON COLD TIMELINE

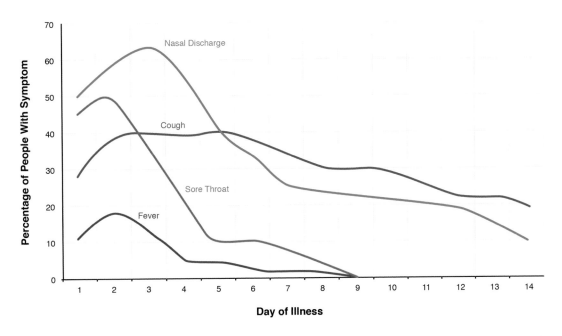

*Gwaltney JM, JAMA 1967; 202:494-498*

**Not only will your child catch six to eight colds a year or more, but each cold will typically take at least two weeks or longer to resolve.**

Fever will usually resolve within three to five days, but it is also not unusual for a fever to last seven to nine days. To be cautious, though, any fever lasting longer than three days should be evaluated by a doctor to make sure there is not a secondary infection brewing.

In other words, although a fever may just be caused by a cold virus by itself, there is a chance that a prolonged fever is representative of a cold that is becoming further complicated by an ear infection, a sinus infection, or pneumonia.

Sore throats will typically resolve in five to seven days. A sore throat that is worsening over time or lasting longer than five days may need to be seen by a doctor.

Congestion and coughs will typically take one to two weeks or longer to improve; however, it is not unusual for a cough to last three to six weeks with a single cold. If a cough is lasting longer than two to three weeks and does not sound like it is improving, it may be worthwhile to have a doctor listen to the lungs to make sure there are no asthma-like issues present.

However, if there are no signs of asthma, there is little that can be done for prolonged coughing. If asthma issues are actually complicating the cold, there are some things that should be done to help control the cough and improve the breathing (see see page 91 for more details).

Remember—**with the common cold, time is the great healer!**

# EXPECT MULTIPLE COLDS PER WINTER

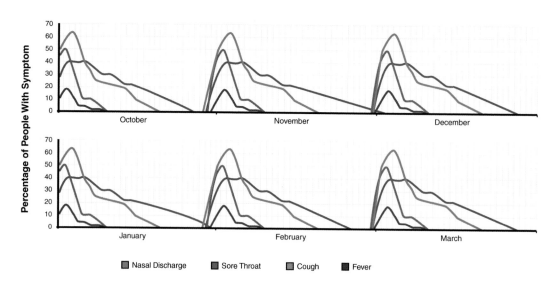

Gwaltney JM, JAMA 1967; 202:494-498

Most children will catch one cold per month during the winter months, typically starting in October and lasting until March. It may seem like your child is a perpetual mucus-producing, coughing machine for nearly six months straight, with just an occasional break from symptoms here and there. Believe it or not, that is pretty typical!

**It is safe to estimate that your child will spend 80 percent of the wintertime with a cough, congestion or both, especially in the first few years of life.** (And you, as the parent, may also feel like you are sick for much of those first few winters!)

A good number of children will suffer from several ear infections as well. While colds cannot be treated, most ear infections can. When an ear infection (see Chapter 5) is suspected, the child should be seen by the doctor. It is also important to be on the lookout for pneumonias and asthma-like issues. Each of these complications and their specific symptoms will be discussed in later chapters.

# THREE REASONS FOR BACK-TO-BACK FEVERS

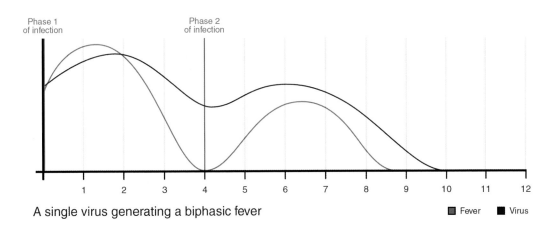

A single virus generating a biphasic fever

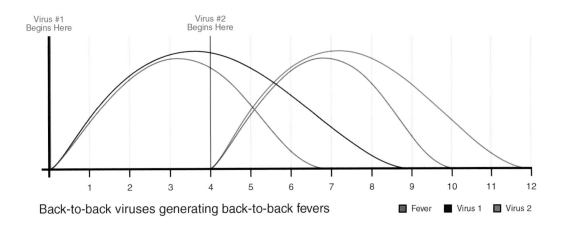

Back-to-back viruses generating back-to-back fevers

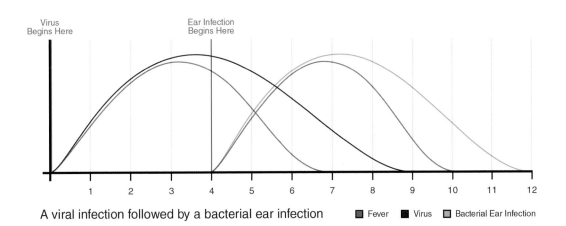

A viral infection followed by a bacterial ear infection

Children will regularly have fevers throughout their life. However, some children may occasionally have back-to-back fevers, when a fever starts, appears to resolve, and then comes roaring back.

There are three typical scenarios which can explain this phenomenon:

The first scenario is one in which a virus attacks the body and, as the immune system begins to defeat the virus, the fever begins to recede; however, the virus then makes a comeback, triggering a second fever. Eventually, the immune system will conquer the virus and the fever will fully resolve.

The second scenario is where a virus attacks the body and, as the immune system begins to defeat the virus, the fever begins to recede; subsequently, a different virus will attack the body and trigger a second fever. Eventually, the immune system will conquer both viruses and the fever will fully resolve.

The third scenario is where a virus attacks the body and, as the immune system begins to defeat the virus, the fever begins to recede; subsequently, a *bacterial* infection (following the initial viral infection) triggers a second fever. Eventually, the immune system will conquer the virus (the bacteria will usually require antibiotics) and the fever will fully resolve.

Generally speaking, any child with back-to-back fevers should be seen by the doctor to ensure a bacterial complication is not settling in. Ear infections, sinus infections, and pneumonias caused by bacteria often require antibiotics and close follow-up care.

## WITH A COMMON COLD, APPETITE LOSS IS TEMPORARY AND COMMON

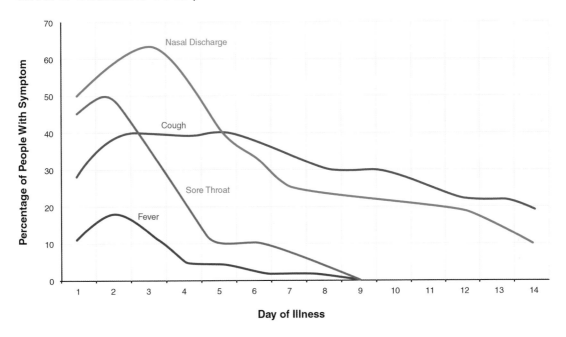

Gwaltney JM, JAMA 1967; 202:494-498

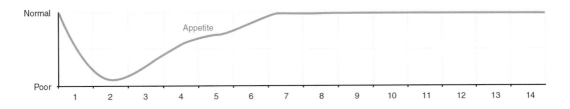

A loss of appetite will accompany most illnesses. It takes energy to digest food; when your child is sick, their body will purposefully stop eating so that it does not have to use energy on the digestive process.

The body has plenty of fat reserves that can temporarily provide energy for the body. The saved energy from not having to digest food will be used to help fight the invading germs. This allows the immune system to more efficiently and rapidly defeat the invading germs.

**With most illnesses, a drop in appetite is to be expected, and is not worrisome as long as the child continues to drink plenty of fluids and is playful and interactive.** However, if a decrease in appetite is also accompanied by a decrease in playfulness and a decrease in interaction, the child should be evaluated for the possibility of a more serious infection.

Appetite will usually inversely mirror fever: As the fever kicks in and rises, appetite will typically diminish, and as the fever fades and the germ is defeated, appetite will return to normal.

## DIFFERENTIATING BETWEEN AN ALLERGY AND THE COMMON COLD

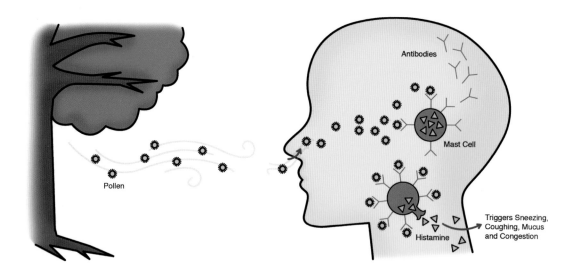

Doctors are often asked how to tell the difference between the common cold and an allergy. The short answer? It's not easy.

Colds and allergies both manifest themselves with mucus, sneezing, cough, and congestion. **In general, colds tend to have more cough and mucus symptoms, and allergies tend to have more sneezing and itchy eye symptoms.**

When a cold virus invades the mucus membranes, it destroys the inner skin cells of the nose and throat, which in turn leads to sneezing, cough, mucus, and congestion. Allergies, on the other hand, occur when allergens (such as pollen) invade the nose and throat, triggering the release of histamine from mast cells, which then leads to sneezing, cough, mucus, and congestion.

Histamine release only occurs with allergies; as such, oral antihistamines will only relieve allergies, and not colds. Thus, one simple way of differentiating between colds and allergies is to give an oral antihistamine daily for 1–2 weeks. If there is an appreciable improvement in symptoms, allergies are likely part (or all) of the underlying problem.

During the wintertime, it is quite possible that children may be afflicted with a cold virus and allergy issues at the same time. When this happens, allergy medications will provide some relief, while the symptoms resulting from the cold will not respond to the allergy medications and will have to run their course over time.

It is important to note that most kids will only develop seasonal allergies after they have been exposed to the same allergen two or three seasons in a row. Hence, **most children younger than 2–3 years of age are unlikely to have allergy issues.**

What to Know Before Seeing Your Pediatrician

# LOCATION MATTERS WITH THE COMMON COLD VIRUS

**Inflammatory Complications**

**Clogging Complications**

As mentioned in the first chapter, location matters! When we think of cold viruses, we think of mucus, cough, and stuffy noses. **However, different types of diseases and symptoms can result based on where the cold virus infects the airway of the child. In other words, the same germ can manifest itself in many different ways, depending on where in the respiratory tract it takes a foothold.**

Picture a classroom, in which all the students pass around the same exact cold virus. Jack's cold virus may deposit in his throat, triggering a viral throat infection (pharyngitis). Sally's cold virus settles in her eyes, precipitating a viral pinkeye (conjunctivitis). Sam's cold virus may block his eustachian tube, which then allows a streptococcus bacteria to fester in his middle ear space, leading to a middle ear infection. The germ remains the same, yet the symptoms differ depending on where the germ makes its home in the body.

The following pictures in this chapter present the different inflammatory complications that a cold virus can elicit. The various clogging complications are discussed in Chapters 5 and 6.

## NASAL INFLAMMATION (RHINITIS)/VIRAL SINUS INFECTION (SINUSITIS)

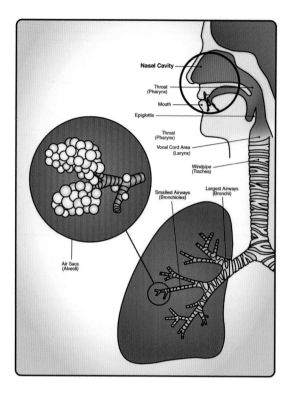

If the cold virus invades the nasal cavity area, the result is nasal inflammation (rhinitis), or what is better known as the **common cold**. **Common colds are characterized by cough, sneezing, runny nose, sore throat, congestion, and fever.**

The cold virus can also invade nearby sinuses (not shown) and trigger a viral sinus infection. Viral sinus infections are far more common than bacterial sinus infections. Unlike a bacterial sinus infection (discussed in Chapter 6), a viral sinus infection does *not* require antibiotics.

Green mucus is triggered by an enzyme called myeloperoxidase and is present with both viral and bacterial infections. **As such, the presence of green mucus is a poor criteria in determining whether antibiotics are needed or not.**

# THROAT INFECTION (PHARYNGITIS)

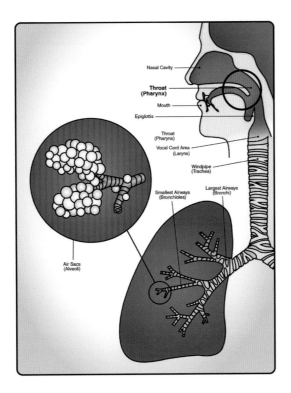

If the cold virus invades the throat area, the result is a **sore throat (pharyngitis),** which often accompanies a common cold. Throat infections caused by a cold virus do not require antibiotics, unlike a strep throat (streptococcal phayrngitis), which does.

**Approximately 85 percent of throat infections are caused by viruses, which means they are far more common than a strep throat infection.** A viral throat infection will heal on its own, but may benefit from gargling with salt water several times a day as needed; otherwise, only supportive care is needed.

Collectively, rhinitis, sinusitis, and pharyngitis are known as **upper respiratory infections**.

# CROUP/LARYNGITIS

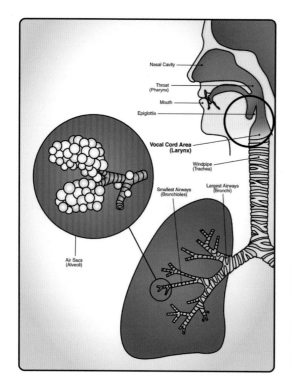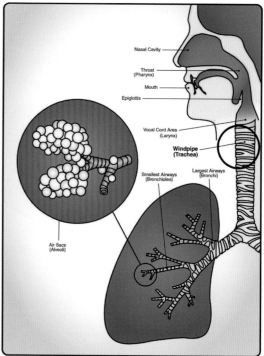

If the cold virus invades the vocal cords or windpipe (trachea), the result is **croup. Croup is characterized by a loud, barky cough. Although croup can look and sound quite dangerous, it rarely is.**

Croup will often produce a stridor breathing sound in the child which mimics wheezing. Stridor is a high-pitched, musical breathing noise heard with inspiration of the lungs, whereas wheezing is more of a whistling sound heard with expiration of the lungs. **If wheezing is present, it indicates involvement of the lungs, which is more concerning and should be reported to the doctor.**

Croup can be treated with oral steroids at the doctor's office to help decrease the inflammation in the vocal cords and windpipe. Home remedies include giving the child a 15-minute steam bath, or stepping outside with the child for a short walk. Most kids quickly improve from croup, with minimal intervention being needed.

Another symptom of the vocal cords being invaded is **laryngitis**, which is characterized by a loss of voice. Laryngitis will resolve in time and requires little intervention other than resting the vocal cords.

# BRONCHITIS/BRONCHIOLITIS

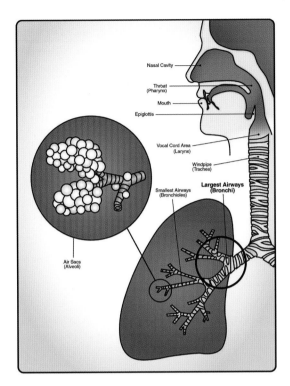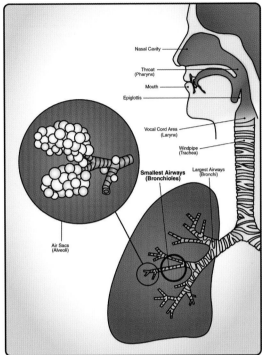

If the cold virus migrates all the way down into the lungs, it can infect and inflame the airways. Large airways are called bronchi, and when they are infected, it is called **bronchitis**. Bronchitis is more common in adults. Small airways are called bronchioles, and when they are infected it is called **bronchiolitis**. Bronchiolitis is more common in young children younger than 2 years of age.

When the airways become infected, wheezing often accompanies the mucus and inflammation of the airway walls. **Imagine the same mucus and stuffiness you feel in your nose happening further down in the airways of your lungs.**

Bronchitis and bronchiolitis are almost always caused by viral infections, yet doctors often over-prescribe antibiotics for these illnesses. Unfortunately, this will not help. Asthma medications (such as steroids and inhalers) are also prescribed by doctors, but provide limited benefits, and only help when the child actually has an underlying asthma problem.

Similar to the common cold, the main problem with bronchiolitis is the damage to the airways caused by the virus itself. Full recovery can take weeks or even months. In young children, hospitalization may be necessary for observation purposes and supportive care (such as oxygen).

If a child is displaying labored breathing or decreasing activity, they should be evaluated by a doctor. Most kids will recover and return back to normal with time, but be prepared for a very long period of coughing.

As a side note, the respiratory synctial virus (RSV) is the most notorious of the bronchiolitis-causing germs, but it only comprises 25 percent of cases, with other cold viruses rounding out the rest. Whether bronchiolitis is triggered by RSV or a different virus, the symptoms and treatment are the same as described above.

## VIRAL PNEUMONIA

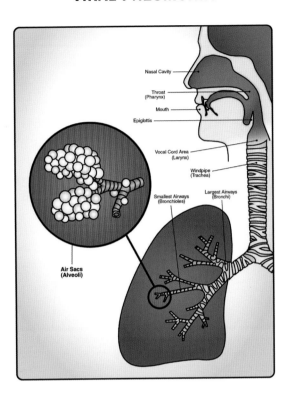

If the virus makes it all the way down into the air sacs of the lung (known as alveoli), a **viral pneumonia** can develop. Viral pneumonia can be cumbersome, and even dangerous in severe cases; however, the majority of cases are not, and most will resolve with time.

Like bronchiolitis, a severe case of viral pneumonia may require hospitalization for the purposes of observation and supportive care. **If a child is displaying labored breathing (appearing as if they just ran a mile) or decreasing activity, they need to be evaluated by a doctor.**

A bacterial pneumonia (discussed in Chapter 6) is more concerning than a viral pneumonia, and must be treated with antibiotics. Bacterial pneumonias will also display labored breathing and decreasing activity. A good physical exam and/or a chest x-ray (although often not needed) can differentiate between a viral and bacterial cause of pneumonia.

# THE THREE ZONES OF THE AIRWAYS

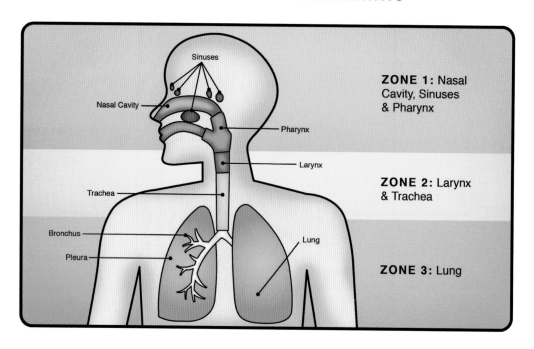

| Zone 1: Upper airways | Nasal cavity, sinuses and pharynx (throat) | Common cold (rhinitis), viral sinus infection and sore throat |
|---|---|---|
| Zone 2: Middle airways | Larynx and trachea (windpipe) | Croup and laryngitis |
| Zone 3: Lower airways | Lungs (bronchi, bronchioles and alveoli) | Bronchitis/bronchiolitis and viral pneumonia |

For a doctor evaluating a child with a respiratory virus, the most important distinction is to determine whether the infection is affecting the upper/middle airways and/or the lower airways. **An infection involving the lower airways (Zone 3) is always more concerning, because compromised lungs may lead to life-threatening complications and as such may require oxygen supplementation and/or closer monitoring in a hospital.** A child with an upper/middle airway issue (Zones 1 and 2) will typically get better on their own, and generally do not need to be seen by a doctor other than for reassurance purposes (and oral steroids for croup).

There are two clear signs that a child's lower airways are becoming involved:

1.  **Retractions:** With each breath, the chest will appear as if it is sinking just below the neckline and/or under the ribcage. The child will breathe as if they just ran a mile. A few minutes of retractions are not too worrisome, but sustained retractions for one hour or more warrant a call or visit to the doctor.

2.  **Increased Breathing Rate:** Count the number of breaths over one minute. If the child is breathing faster than the age-appropriate normal rate for a period of one hour or more, call the doctor.

| Age | Normal Respiratory Rate |
| --- | --- |
| Normal rates: Infant (birth–1 year) | 30–60 |
| Toddler (1–3 years) | 24–40 |
| Preschooler (3–6 years) | 22–34 |
| School-age (6–12 years) | 18–30 |

Other concerning signs of lower airway involvement include flaring of the nostrils, grunting noises, wheezing noises and changes in the color of complexion (pale, gray, or blue).

Bear in mind that the above chart does not include the bacterial infections that can result from a clogging complication of any of the above viral infections. Refer back to page 51 for a better overview of the different bacterial manifestations that can follow a viral infection.

# TAKE-HOME POINTS

★ There are no effective cough and cold medications for children.

★ There are two major categories of common cold complications: inflammatory complications and clogging complications.

★ Most kids will catch at least six to eight colds per year.

★ Coughing is more copious at nighttime due to poor drainage of mucus when lying down.

★ Full recovery from the common cold can take two weeks or longer.

★ For a common cold, time is the great healer.

★ Back-to-back fevers should be evaluated by a doctor.

★ Allergies and colds are similar in appearance, but an antihistamine trial may help discriminate between the two.

★ Location matters! Depending on where the cold virus invades, different symptoms and diseases can occur.

★ Think of the airway in three zones: upper, middle, and lower. Cold viruses can cause unique complications in each zone.

★ Lower airway infections are cause for concern, and the sustained presence of retractions and/or increased respiratory rate warrant a call to the doctor.

The cold virus is ubiquitous, making it impossible to avoid during wintertime. Children will catch their fair share of cold viruses no matter how careful and hygienic they are. Depending on where the virus invades, different symptoms and diseases will occur.

Most inflammatory complications of the cold virus will require minimal intervention and will typically resolve with time and supportive care.

Should a child present with labored breathing, decreased activity, or back-to-back fevers, a visit to the doctor is warranted. For the most part, most colds and their inflammatory complications can be handled at home with some tender loving care and time.

What to Know Before Seeing Your Pediatrician

# Chapter 5

# EAR INFECTIONS

THE MOST frequent clogging complication of the common cold is a **middle ear infection** (also known as an inner ear infection or otitis media). If your child is still acting fussy several days after a cold infection has occurred, or if a new fever kicks in, there is a good chance that they may have a middle ear infection.

Pulling on the ears may also signal an ear infection, but only if other symptoms are also present. Children will pull on their ears for all sorts of reasons, including the most common one—because they can!

**Middle ear infections are the most common reason for young children to receive oral antibiotics**.

Most middle ear infections will need to be seen by the doctor. Unfortunately, kids who get middle ear infections are prone to getting them quite frequently, some of which is due to the anatomy of the Eustachian tube. Fortunately, there are good options available to help treat and contain the number of middle ear infections children have.

# MIDDLE EAR INFECTIONS AND OUTER EAR INFECTIONS OCCUR IN DIFFERENT PLACES

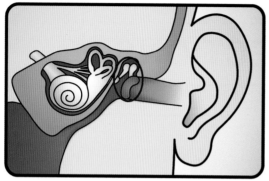
Where middle ear infections occur

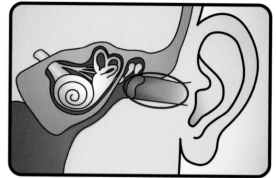
Where outer ear infections occur

**It is important to note that there are two different types of ear infections, which occur in different parts of the ear: One is a middle ear infection, and the other is an outer ear infection.**

The middle ear infection (also known as an inner ear infection or otitis media) occurs in the middle ear space that sits *behind* the eardrum.

The outer ear infection (also known as otitis externa or swimmer's ear infection) occurs in the outer ear canal that sits *in front of* the eardrum. Anatomically, these are two different types of infections.

Water in the ear canal can trigger a swimmer's ear infection, but it cannot trigger a middle ear infection. Middle ear infections happen when the Eustachian tube becomes clogged, as explained later in this chapter.

## HOW A SWIMMER'S EAR INFECTION HAPPENS

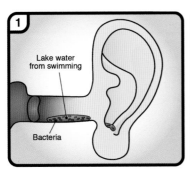
**1** Lake water from swimming — Bacteria

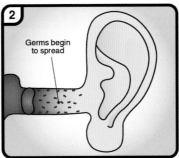
**2** Germs begin to spread

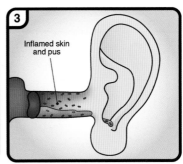
**3** Inflamed skin and pus

Swimmer's ear infections typically occur when sweat or water become trapped in the outer ear canal. Bacteria may be present in the incoming water, or they may already reside in the ear canal as colonized germs.

**When water stagnates in the ear, it provides a moist environment, making it easier for bacteria to fester and rapidly multiply, leading to a swimmer's ear infection.** Bath water is a rare culprit as it quickly evaporates from the ear canal.

Usually, the treatment of swimmer's ear infections only requires antibiotic ear drops, placed in the outside canal of the offending ear for five to seven days. If there is a heavy amount of inflammation, an oral antibiotic may also be necessary.

# HOW A MIDDLE EAR INFECTION HAPPENS

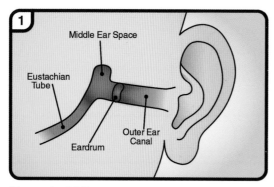

Normal middle ear space

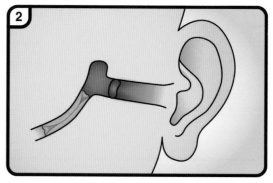

A cold virus creates mucus, blocking the Eustachian tube

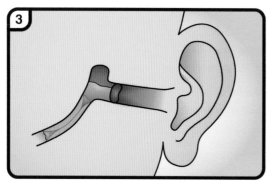

Fluid becomes trapped in the middle ear

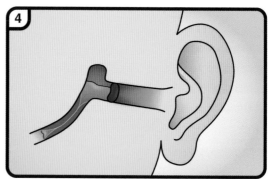

The fluid becomes infected with a bacteria

The process of developing a middle ear infection, on the other hand, is a bit more complicated:

1. The middle ear space typically drains via the Eustachian tube into the throat. **As long as the Eustachian tube stays open, middle ear infections will not form.**

2. When a child catches a viral cold infection, much like how the nose becomes swollen and congested with mucus, the Eustachian tube also becomes swollen and congested with mucus.

3. Fluid regularly secreted by the inner skin cells of the middle ear that would typically drain via the Eustachian tube becomes trapped in the middle ear space.

4. Bacteria then fester and multiply in the trapped water, leading to a middle ear infection.

What to Know Before Seeing Your Pediatrician

## THE BACTERIA THAT TRIGGER MIDDLE EAR INFECTIONS ARE ALREADY COLONIZED IN THE BODY

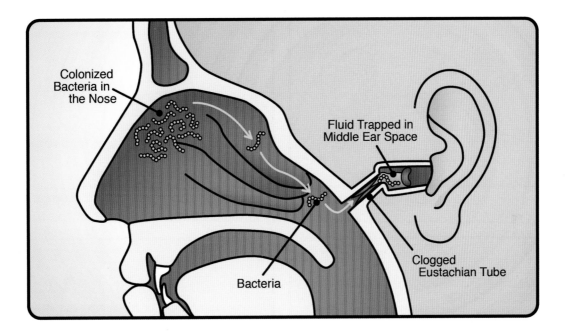

**The bacteria that trigger a middle ear infection may already be colonized in the middle ear space or else may come over from colonization residing in the nose, or any part of the nose/throat area.**

Colonized bacteria will not trigger disease unless they have a nice environment in which to multiply, such as trapped water or mucus. Once they find a home, the bacteria will wildly proliferate, leading to inflammation, pus, pressure, pain, and fever.

Because clogging complications are a result of a complex, multistep process and are often triggered by self-colonized bacteria, they are not considered contagious. The underlying cold virus that triggers the mucus and congestion is contagious, but the clogging complication itself is not.

Note that a middle ear infection may also be due solely to a virus, without bacteria being involved. Just as bacteria can proliferate in an enclosed middle ear space, viruses can do this as well. It is less common for middle ear infections to only be caused by a virus; however, when this happens, antibiotics are not needed.

Differentiating between a viral and bacterial middle ear infection is not easy, and as most middle ear infections *are* bacterial, doctors will generally err on the side of treating with antibiotics, especially if the child is having noticeable pain.

## AFTER ORAL ANTIBIOTICS, REOPENING OF THE EUSTACHIAN TUBE CAN TAKE DAYS/WEEKS

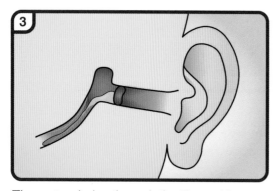

Oral antibiotics penetrate the middle ear

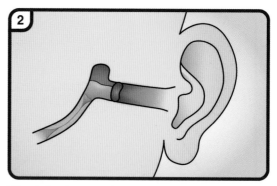

The infection resolves, leaving behind fluid in the middle ear space

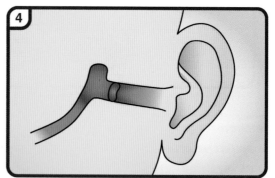

The water drains through the Eustachian tube as it unclogs over time

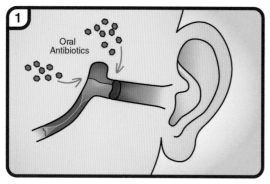

The middle ear returns back to normal

Once a middle ear infection occurs, oral antibiotics will generally be necessary to treat the infection and to help control any pain or fussiness. Antibiotic ear drops will not penetrate through the ear drum into the middle ear space and are therefore not helpful (unless the child has tubes in place, or the eardrum perforates—both scenarios are discussed later in this chapter).

However, because some of the pain is from inflammation of the eardrum, pain drops (which are different from antibiotic ear drops) placed in the ear canal can help. Acetaminophen and ibuprofen can also be given to help control discomfort and pain.

After a middle ear infection is appropriately treated with antibiotics, the bacteria in the middle ear space will usually be eradicated and the child will feel much better, but the Eustachian tube will often remain clogged. **This means that fluid will remain trapped in the middle ear space**

**for days, or even weeks after the ear infection is treated.** This persistence of fluid sets the child up for additional middle ear infections. Over time, the Eustachian tube will eventually reopen, allowing the trapped fluid to finally drain.

Unfortunately, there are no medications that work well to unclog a blocked Eustachian tube. As you might guess by now, in general, your best option is to give it time.

# THE EUSTACHIAN TUBE GROWS IN SIZE AND BECOMES MORE VERTICAL AS KIDS GET OLDER

Baby

Adult

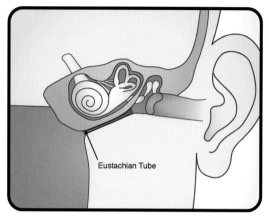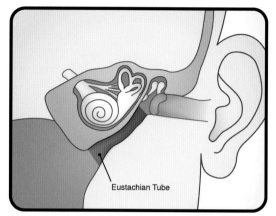

There are several reasons why babies and children get more middle ear infections than adults, but the biggest one is the anatomy of the ear's drainage pipe, the Eustachian tube.

**In a baby, the Eustachian tube has a narrow diameter and lies nearly horizontal, which makes it harder for fluid to drain from the middle ear space to the throat. As a child grows bigger, the Eustachian tubes become wider in diameter and begin to move vertically downward, improving drainage and thus reducing the risk of middle ear infections.**

Anyone who has ever flown on a plane has experienced a blocked Eustachian tube. The pressure changes that occur on takeoff and landing lead to short-term blockage of the Eustachian tubes. This can be mildly discomforting until the tube reopens. Swallowing often helps to relieve the blockage.

In most kids, the transition to healthy drainage of the Eustachian tubes will occur around 2 years of age. Some children may experience this later.

Some families have genetically small Eustachian tubes that make them especially prone to middle ear infections. These kids will be frequent fliers in the office and will often require multiple courses of antibiotics each year.

Many of these kids will end up benefiting from pressure equalizing tubes (PETs), which are discussed later in this chapter. A case-by-case discussion with the doctor is the best way to decide which child will benefit from having PET surgery.

What to Know Before Seeing Your Pediatrician

## THE TYPICAL TIMELINE OF A MIDDLE EAR INFECTION BEGINS WITH A COMMON COLD

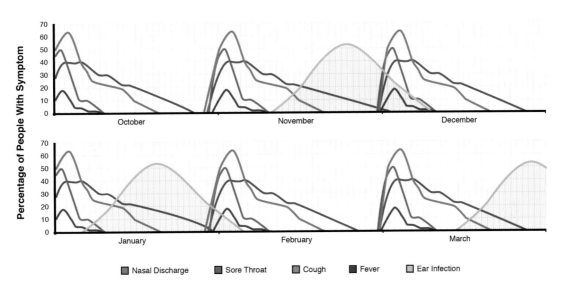

Gwaltney JM. JAMA 1967: 202:494-498

**The typical timeline of a middle ear infection begins with a common cold.** As discussed earlier, this leads to mucus blocking the Eustachian tube, which leads to water backing up in the middle ear space, which then becomes infected with bacteria.

The jump from a cold to an ear infection can sometimes develop over a short period of one to two days, but it may also play out over one to two weeks. It is quite common for a child to be seen by a doctor and receive the diagnosis of a viral cold without a middle ear infection, only to develop one 24 hours later.

A typical child prone to middle ear infections (due to small Eustachian tubes) may develop four to six (or more) middle ear infections in a single year. Generally speaking, each ear infection will require a course of antibiotics to treat it.

There is a possibility that the repeated use of the same antibiotic will render it ineffective as the bacteria become resistant to the medication over time. This may necessitate the eventual use of stronger antibiotics. The need for this should be determined on a case-by-case basis, and when possible, the weakest antibiotic that can successfully combat the bacteria should be chosen.

## CHILDREN MAY HAVE FLUID IN THEIR MIDDLE EAR SPACE
## INTERMITTENTLY THROUGHOUT THE WINTER

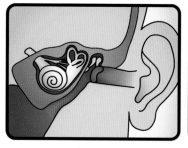 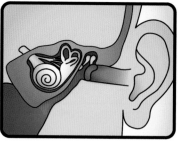 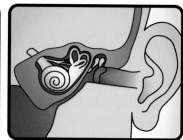

Large                    Medium                    Small

Since most kids will catch multiple colds during the wintertime, the majority of young children (4 years and younger) will have some fluid in the middle ear space intermittently throughout the cold season.

**The smaller the Eustachian tube is, the more likely it is to become clogged.**

Children who are lucky enough to inherit large Eustachian tubes will rarely have fluid in their middle ear space. Those who inherit medium-sized Eustachian tubes will have fluid off and on throughout the winter. And those who inherit small Eustachian tubes will be afflicted with multiple middle ear infections and will have constant fluid in their middle ear space throughout the entire winter.

The longer that fluid is trapped in the middle ear space, the more likely it is that a middle ear infection will occur. It is possible, though, that some kids will have fluid trapped in the middle ear space for weeks (or sometimes months) without actually developing a middle ear infection.

Conversely, it is also possible for trapped fluid to develop into a middle ear infection overnight.

Parents often ask if they can preempt an ear infection by treating a child who has fluid in the middle ear with antibiotics before an actual middle ear infection settles in. Studies have shown that this does not reduce the overall number of middle ear infections. Additionally, it may make matters worse by increasing the odds of antibiotic-resistant bacteria in future middle ear infections.

In deciding when to use antibiotics, it is best to cross that bridge when you actually get there.

## AFTER A MIDDLE EAR INFECTION, THE EUSTACHIAN TUBE NEEDS TIME TO RETURN TO BASELINE

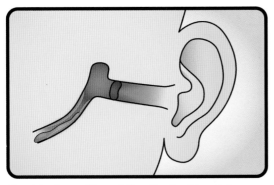

Residual swelling of the Eustachian tube

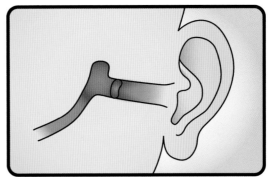

Normal Eustachian tube

**Once a single middle ear infection occurs, it takes time for the swelling of the Eustachian tube to fully resolve and get back to its baseline draining ability.**

A middle ear infection may occur even in spite of genetically large Eustachian tubes. Despite proper treatment, the ear infection then leaves behind residual swelling within the Eustachian tube, rendering the tube narrower, and thus easier for a second blockage and a subsequent ear infection to occur.

This is why a child, who has never had a single ear infection in the first two years of life, may all of a sudden have three ear infections back-to-back-to-back. This is very commonly seen and is not a cause for alarm.

Once the Eustachian tube is able to fully recuperate and return to its normal size, it will again drain appropriately, and the chain of ear infections should subside. It usually takes several months of being free from any new colds for the Eustachian tube to fully recover; as such, back-to-back ear infections typically occur during the wintertime, with relief coming in the springtime.

## IN CHILDREN OLDER THAN 2 YEARS, THE MIDDLE EAR INFECTION MAY RESOLVE WITHOUT ANTIBIOTICS

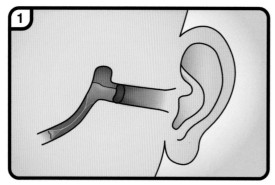

Middle ear infection is present

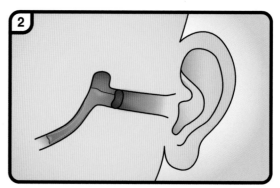

Over time, the Eustachian tube unclogs

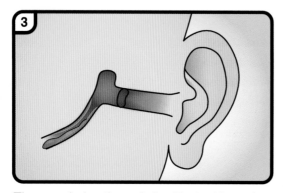

The pus drains through the Eustachian tube

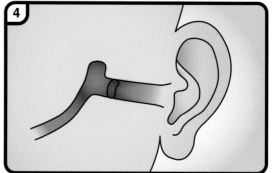

The middle ear returns back to normal

In children older than 2 years who do not have a chronic history of middle ear infections, antibiotics may not be necessary to treat the middle ear infection.

**In approximately 80 percent of children older than 2 years who have a middle ear infection, the Eustachian tube will spontaneously open, allowing the pus to drain from the middle ear and heal on its own.** This is akin to a pimple that pops and then heals. In 20 percent of kids, however, this will not happen and the middle ear infection will require oral antibiotics.

If there is a heavy history of past or recent middle ear infections, there is a lower likelihood that the infection will resolve without treatment. In general, the more pain and discomfort a child has, the more likely that treatment should be initiated. A doctor's examination coupled with the child's medical history can help determine whether or not to treat with antibiotics.

What to Know Before Seeing Your Pediatrician

# RUPTURED MIDDLE EAR INFECTION

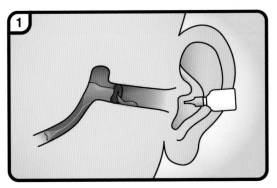

Pressure from the middle ear infection leads to a rupture of the eardrum

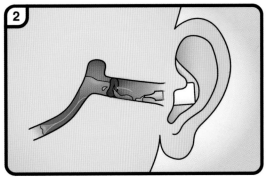

Antibiotic ear drops are placed in the canal and enter the middle ear space through the hole in the eardrum

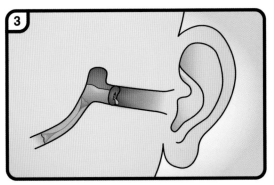

The infection resolves, leaving behind fluid in the middle ear space

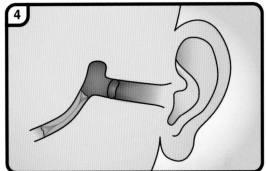

Over time, the eardrum heals

**Sometimes, a middle ear infection will create so much pressure in the middle ear space that the eardrum itself will rupture.** Pus will then leak from the middle ear space out into the ear canal. Children will often be in pain prior to the rupture occurring, but will experience significant relief after the rupture occurs.

Treatment options vary. At times, doctors will treat the infection with just ear antibiotic drops (as shown). Other times, doctors will do both ear antibiotic drops and oral antibiotics, particularly if there is a large amount of pus present in the outer ear canal. In general, treating with drops alone is adequate, but this should be determined on a case-by-case basis.

Even after the infection is appropriately treated, the Eustachian tube will often remain clogged, setting up the child for additional middle ear infections. In time though, the Eustachian tube should open up and the ear will return back to its normal state.

# PRESSURE EQUALIZING TUBES (PET) OR EAR TUBES

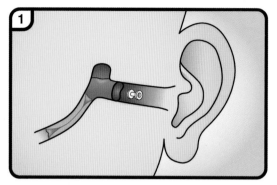

Water is trapped in the middle ear space

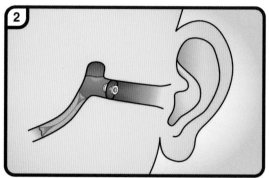

PET is placed in the eardrum

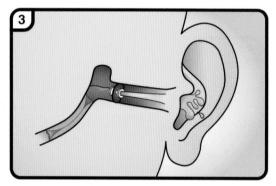

Water exits through the PET

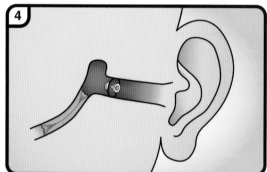

The clogging of the Eustachian tube may persist indefinitely

**In children who get frequent middle ear infections and have had four or more in a 12-month period, pressure equalizing tubes (PET) may be recommended by the doctor.** Not all kids who get frequent ear infections will need PETs. Although PET placement is a safe procedure, it does require general anesthesia. As such, there is some medical risk in undergoing the procedure, and the decision to have surgery is best made on a case-by-case basis.

The PET works by placing an artificial drain within the eardrum. When the Eustachian tube becomes blocked, the presence of the PET allows water in the middle ear space to drain out via an alternative pathway, thus preventing a middle ear infection from occurring.

Both allergies and colds can lead to mucus and congestion, which in turn can clog the Eustachian tube, triggering a middle ear infection—although colds are by far the more common cause, especially in kids younger than 2 years of age. Some doctors may initially recommend allergy medications in an attempt to alleviate the blockage of the Eustachian tubes before fully committing to PET surgery.

## MIDDLE EAR INFECTION IN SPITE OF A PET

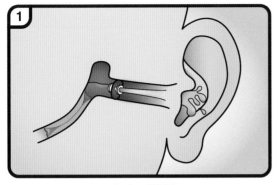

Water exits through the PET

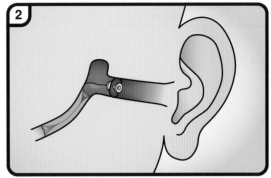

Some water remains in the middle ear space

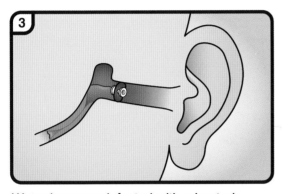

Water becomes infected with a bacteria

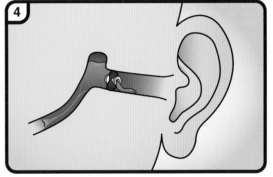

Pus leaks through the PET

Although PETs will significantly reduce the number of middle ear infections, they are not 100 percent effective.

**At times, even with PETs in place, enough fluid can still become trapped behind the middle ear space to allow bacteria to mount an infection.**

This does not happen often, and most kids after having PET surgery will see a significant improvement in their number of ear infections. But should a middle ear infection with a PET in place occur, it will be substantially less painful to a child because of the release of pressure via the PET. Treatment is also easier as antibiotic ear drops can be used to directly treat the infection via the PET.

## EARWAX BLOCKING THE PET

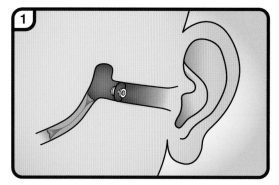

PET is open but the Eustachian tube is blocked

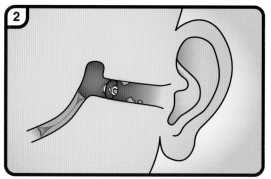

PET becomes blocked with ear wax

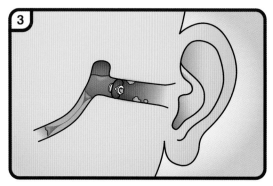

Water is trapped in middle ear space

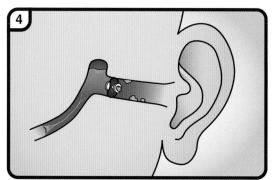

Water becomes infected with a bacteria

**Another way a middle ear infection can occur with PETs is if the tube itself becomes blocked with earwax or debris.**

Once the PET is blocked, water can accumulate in the middle ear space and a middle ear infection can occur.

With a simple fix, a surgeon can suction out the offending wax so that the PET drains appropriately again.

Using cotton-tipped applicators to clean the outside of the ear canal (the area that is visible) can help keep the ear clean. However, it is not a good idea to use the applicators to clean the inside of the canal as it will typically push the ear wax further inward and possibly lead to blockage of the PET.

**What to Know Before Seeing Your Pediatrician**

## A DRAINING MIDDLE EAR INFECTION WITH PETS CAN BE TREATED WITH JUST ANTIBIOTIC DROPS

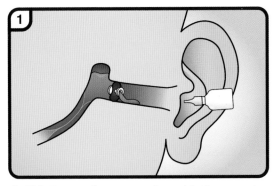

Antibiotic ear drops are placed in the canal

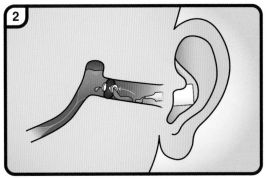

The drops enter the middle ear space through the PET

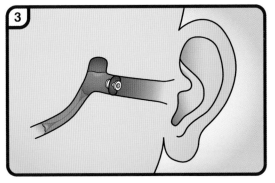

The infection resolves, leaving behind fluid in the middle ear space

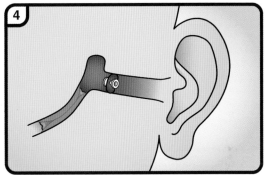

Over time, the water drains through the PET

**Treatment of a draining middle ear infection with a PET in place can usually be accomplished with just the use of antibiotic ear drops.**

Drainage confirms that the PET is not blocked. However, if the PET *is* blocked, and little or no drainage is present, an oral antibiotic may be necessary.

A doctor may also recommend oral antibiotics if the drainage is quite thick and there is concern whether or not the drops will penetrate deep enough into the middle ear space.

# PETS WILL NATURALLY FALL OUT WITH TIME

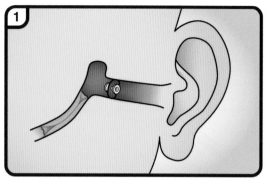

The clogging of the Eustachian tube will often persist despite the placement of the PETs

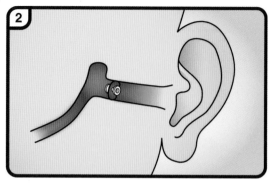

The Eustachian tubes should unclog over time

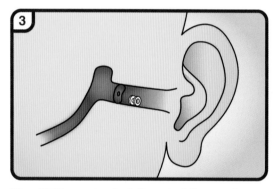

The PET eventually falls out of the eardrum

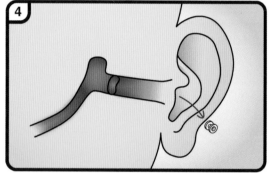

Over time, the PET falls out of the ear canal

**Over time, PETs will naturally be pushed out of the eardrum (due to the repeated turnover of the eardrum skin cells) and will then eventually fall out of the ear canal on their own.**

Once the PET falls out, the hole in the eardrum will naturally heal and close on its own.

At times, if the PET becomes embedded in wax or remains in the eardrum longer than two to three years, the ENT (ear, nose and throat) surgeon may need to extract the PET.

The typical PET will function effectively and stay intact within the eardrum for six to 18 months.

In children with genetically small Eustachian tubes who get frequent ear infections, multiple sets of PETs may be needed over the first few years of life.

What to Know Before Seeing Your Pediatrician

## TYPICALLY, THE BEST TIME TO GET PETS IS THE BEGINNING OF THE COLD SEASON

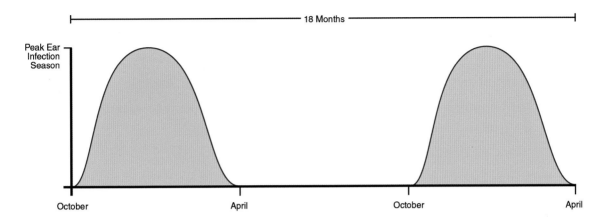

Because most ear infections (triggered by colds) happen in the fall and wintertime, children will benefit most from PETs during the winter season.

**As most PETs will only stay in the eardrum six to 18 months, it is best (if possible) to have the PETs placed right before the cold season starts.**

This will allow for the greatest possibility that two winter seasons of colds and potential ear infections will be alleviated by the placement of a single set of PETs. Of course, having the surgery in the early fall is not always possible or reasonable. Ultimately, the optimal timing of the surgery should be determined on a case-by-case basis.

# TAKE-HOME POINTS

★ Middle ear infections are different from swimmer's ear infections.

★ Middle ear infections are a result of a poorly draining Eustachian tube.

★ Bacteria that trigger middle ear infections often come from the individual's own body.

★ The Eustachian tube gets wider and more vertical with time, allowing for better drainage.

★ Middle ear infections typically follow a viral cold.

★ Allergies are an uncommon trigger for a middle ear infection, especially in children younger than 2 years of age.

★ In children older than 2 years, middle ear infections may resolve without antibiotics.

★ PETs can help drain middle ear fluid, preventing middle ear infections.

★ If possible, the optimal placement of PETs is before the cold season begins.

Ear infections are a vexing problem for many kids in the first few years of life. Luckily, as children grow bigger, so do their Eustachian tubes, reducing the set-up for middle ear infections as the tubes become wider and more vertical.

For children whose DNA predisposes them to small Eustachian tubes, PETs (pressure equalizing tubes) can help alleviate the number of ear infections by preventing the trapping of water in the middle ear space.

When a middle ear infection does occur, prompt treatment with antibiotics can help mitigate pain and suffering.

## Chapter 6

# OTHER COMPLICATIONS
# OF THE COMMON COLD

THE COMMON cold virus can lead to a host of issues in children. Some of these issues are clogging complications, such as a middle ear infection (discussed in Chapter 5).

Among the other issues are inflammatory complications. The cold virus produces inflammation in different areas of the body, resulting in pain and discomfort.

A cold virus can also trigger an asthma attack in certain genetically predisposed individuals—a situation that may require medication in order to help control symptoms.

This chapter reviews some of the other clogging and inflammatory complications of the common cold not discussed in Chapters 4 and 5, such as a sinus infection, pneumonia, pinkeye, costochondritis, pleurisy, and asthma. Some of these complications require antibiotics (if bacteria are involved); others will resolve on their own with time, needing only supportive care and pain relief.

# HOW A BACTERIAL SINUS INFECTION HAPPENS

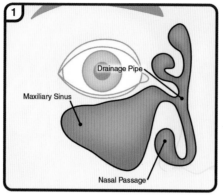

Normal sinus

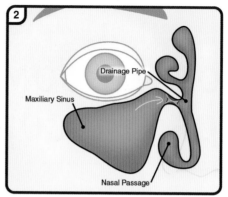

Mucus and inflammation block the drainage pipe

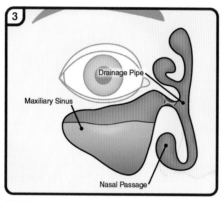

Fluid becomes trapped in the sinus

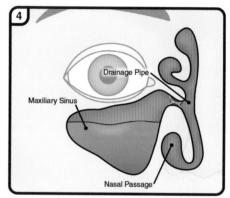

The fluid becomes infected with a bacteria

The sinuses are a system of connected cavities in the skull that help humidify the air we breathe and help enhance our voices.

Sinus infections happen in a similar fashion to a middle ear infection.

1. Each of the sinuses has a drainage pipe. As long as the drainage pipe stays open, an infection should not occur.

2. When a child catches a viral cold infection, the subsequent mucus and inflammation blocks the natural drainage pipe of the sinus.

3. Fluid regularly secreted by the inner skin cells of the sinus then becomes trapped in the sinus area.

4. Bacteria then fester and multiply in the trapped water, leading to a bacterial sinus infection.

## SINUSES DEVELOP IN CHILDREN OVER THE FIRST TEN YEARS OF LIFE

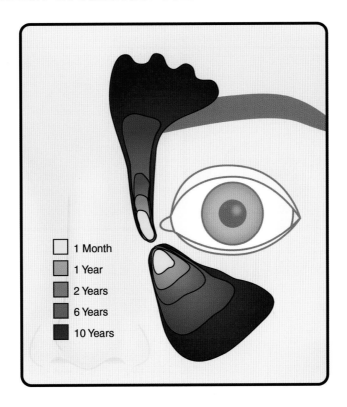

1 Month
1 Year
2 Years
6 Years
10 Years

Sinuses develop in children during their first nine to 10 years of life. **Because children do not have fully developed sinuses like adults, children do not commonly get true bacterial sinus infections.** Even in adults, bacterial sinus infections are over-diagnosed. Most sinus infections only involve a virus, and thus do not require antibiotics.

One common misconception is that green mucus indicates a bacterial sinus infection. Green mucus is caused by an enzyme called myeloperoxidase, which is activated in both bacterial and viral infections. **The presence of green mucus, in and of itself, is *not* a reason to start antibiotics.** Many viral colds and viral sinus infections will produce green mucus, and do not require antibiotics.

Another misconception is that every cold lasting more than 10 days requires antibiotics. *Most* colds will last more than 10 days, and adhering to this misconception will lead to overuse of antibiotics. Indicators of a true bacterial sinus infection are: significant sinus pain, headaches, fever, and nasal drainage of thick, foul-smelling mucus. When a true bacterial sinus infection occurs, antibiotics are necessary.

# HOW PNEUMONIA HAPPENS

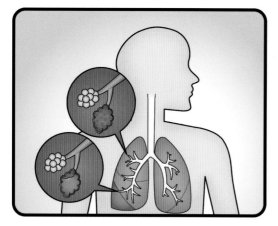 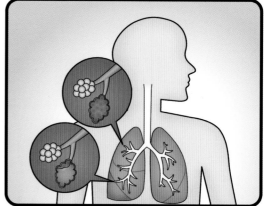

Pneumonias, which are infections of the lungs, also occur in similar fashion to middle ear infections.

The child initially catches a cold, leading to mucus and congestion. The mucus runs down the windpipe and collects in the lung, eventually overwhelming the natural drainage mechanism of the lungs. This leads to fluid getting trapped in the lungs. Eventually, bacteria infect the stagnant fluid and precipitate a bacterial pneumonia.

A bacterial pneumonia is typically preceded by a cold. **The child will appear to be slowly recovering from the cold, when there is a sudden and obvious drop in their activity level. Coughing will sharply increase, and their breathing will appear markedly labored (appearing as if they ran a mile).** If these changes are observed, a doctor's visit is warranted— ASAP.

Like a sinus infection, pneumonia can also be triggered by a virus, without any bacterial involvement. There is also a certain atypical bacteria called Mycoplasma that can trigger a condition known as walking pneumonia. Neither of these pneumonias are as serious as a bacterial pneumonia.

Bacterial pneumonias require antibiotics and could also necessitate hospitalization or even surgery. If untreated, a bacterial pneumonia may lead to large amounts of fluid in the lungs or the formation of pockets of pus. If caught in time, a bacterial pneumonia can be handled with close follow-up care in the doctor's office, and hospitalization and surgery will be avoided. An experienced clinician can diagnose the presence of a bacterial pneumonia without an x-ray, although there are situations when an x-ray is warranted.

Viral pneumonias do not need medication, but may require supportive care (such as oxygen). Walking pneumonias will improve with a certain class of antibiotics known as **macrolides**.

# HOW A BACTERIAL PINKEYE INFECTION HAPPENS

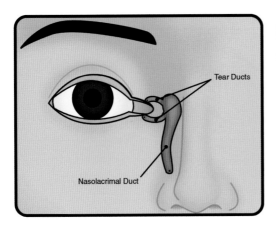

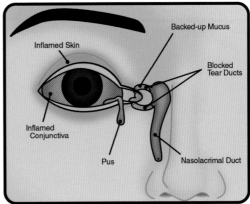

As you might guess, a bacterial pinkeye infection (conjunctivitis) *also* happens in a similar fashion to a middle ear infection.

The child initially catches a cold, leading to mucus and congestion. The mucus blocks the tear ducts that normally drain the eye. Mucus and tears then get backed up in the eye. Eventually, bacteria infect the mucus and backed-up water, leading to a bacterial pinkeye.

Bacterial pinkeye can become serious quickly and should be treated with antibiotic eye drops. **Newer, expensive eye drops are rolled out regularly by pharmaceutical companies, but the older, cheaper antibiotic eye drops generally work well.**

# HOW TO DIFFERENTIATE BETWEEN THE DIFFERENT TYPES OF PINKEYE (BACTERIAL, VIRAL, AND ALLERGIC)

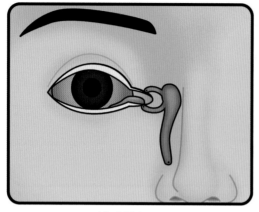

Viral Pinkeye

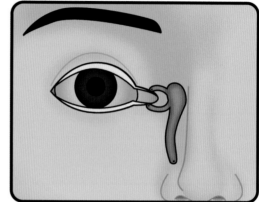

Allergic Pinkeye

Like a sinus infection or pneumonia, some types of pinkeye are triggered by a virus, with no bacterial involvement.

**In fact, viral pinkeye is far more common than bacterial pinkeye, and does not require antibiotic drops.** Like a cold, it will improve over the course of seven to 10 days with no medications.

Allergic pinkeye is also fairly common, but it generally occurs in children older than 2 years of age. Allergic pinkeye can be treated with over-the-counter antihistamine eye drops.

For viral and allergic pinkeye, many doctors will prescribe antibiotic eye drops either unwittingly or prophylactically, to prevent it from evolving into a bacterial infection.

Schools often require children with any version of pinkeye to be on antibiotic eye drops, and do not distinguish between a bacterial, viral, or allergic cause. This can lead to unnecessary prescriptions and purchases of expensive medications.

Bacterial pinkeye should be treated when present. What separates a bacterial pinkeye from the other two is the presence of copious discharge that must be wiped away on an hourly basis. Both viral and allergic pinkeye *will* present with goop in the eye, but this is largely present first thing in the morning; and unlike a bacterial pinkeye, little will accumulate throughout the rest of the day.

Another sign of bacterial pinkeye is swelling and redness of the skin around the eye, which, if left untreated, will worsen with each passing day. Any worsening of symptoms should be seen by a doctor as soon as possible.

# COSTOCHONDRITIS

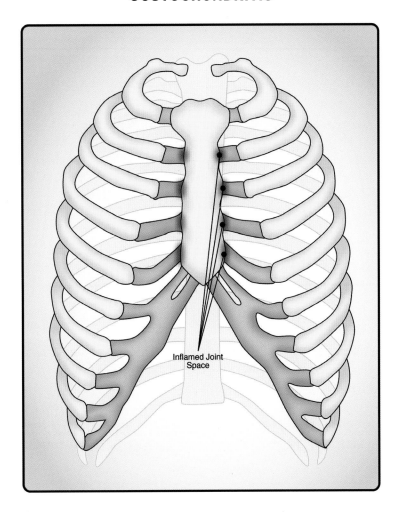

Inflamed Joint Space

A common inflammatory complication of the cold that causes chest pain is **costochondritis**, or inflammation of the joint space between the ribs and the breastplate (sternum).

Costochondritis, unlike previously mentioned clogging complications, is *not* a secondary effect of mucus clogging a drainage pipe. **It is simply triggered by a cold virus migrating to a joint space and causing inflammation, or from inflammation of the joint space as a result of severe bouts of coughing.**

Chest pain will occur with any movement of the upper body, or pressure being placed on the joint space. Like the common cold, this will resolve with time and rest. Pain relievers such as ibuprofen and acetaminophen can be taken to alleviate pain and discomfort.

# PLEURISY

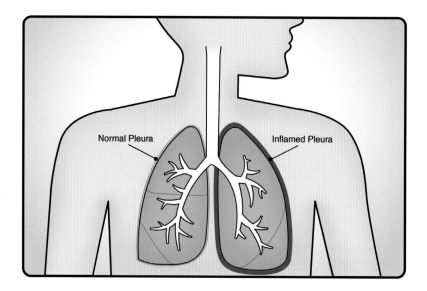

Another inflammatory complication that causes chest pain is known as **pleurisy**, which is the inflammation of the double pleural membranes surrounding your lungs. The pleural membranes are like a sort of plastic wrap surrounding your lungs, which helps to keep them well lubricated and moving easily.

Normally, the double membranes move smoothly against each other as the lung inhales and exhales. However, **when a cold virus invades the pleural membrane, it becomes rough like sandpaper. As the lung inhales and exhales, a sharp pain is felt, almost as if being poked with a sharp object.**

Like the common cold, this will resolve with time and rest. Pain relievers such as ibuprofen and acetaminophen can be taken to alleviate pain and discomfort.

## HOW ASTHMA AFFECTS YOUR LUNGS

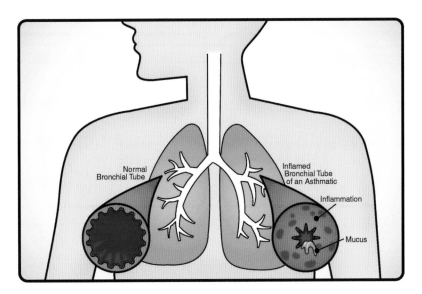

In genetically predisposed individuals, asthma can be a serious complication when triggered by a cold virus. Asthma is a complex disease—one which would require several chapters to explain adequately—but a short summary here can help parents know what to look for. Like bronchitis and bronchiolitis (described in Chapter 4), asthma is essentially an airway issue.

When triggered by a cold virus (which is the most likely scenario, amidst the many other triggers for asthma), the asthmatic airway will become inflamed and filled with mucus, leading to some combination of wheezing, shortness of breath, labored breathing, flaring of the nostrils, and retractions of the chest muscles.

**Unlike bronchitis and bronchiolitis, which can affect any individual, asthma issues usually only affect those people with a genetic predisposition. There is usually a family history of asthma, typically found in mom and/or dad.** Both asthma and bronchitis/bronchiolitis create a narrowing of the airway, and thus appear similarly; as such, it is difficult even for an experienced doctor to tell them apart.

Asthma medications can help control asthma, but will not make much of a difference in a child with bronchitis or bronchiolitis. Asthma medications are typically safe, so it is reasonable to attempt a trial of these medications to see if a child responds.

If there *is* a good response, the good news is that there are medications that can help. The bad news is that the child may have asthma (or at least a mild form of it). If there is a poor response, the good news is that the child likely does not have asthma. The bad news is that there are likely no medications that will help alleviate their immediate symptoms.

# HOW TO PROPERLY USE AN INHALER BY ADDING A SPACER

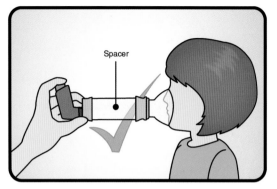
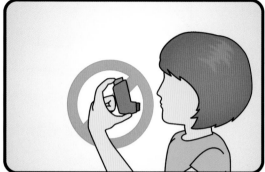

There are two basic mechanisms by which asthma medications can be delivered: the nebulizer (not shown) and the inhaler with spacer (shown above).

Because of its portability, cost savings, and time efficiency, the inhaler (with spacer) is generally preferred over the nebulizer. However, both are equally effective.

**It is important to emphasize that when using an inhaler, a spacer must be used for the medicine to turn into a mist, which can then more easily reach the lungs.** Without the spacer, a good portion of the medication will be deposited in the mouth and will be lost.

# PREVENTATIVE MEDICATIONS VS. RESCUE MEDICATIONS

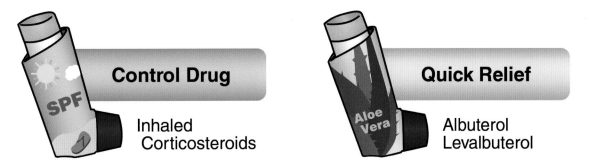

**Control Drug**
Inhaled Corticosteroids

**Quick Relief**
Albuterol Levalbuterol

There are two basic groups of asthma medications: **preventative medicines** and **rescue medicines**.

The rescue medicine that is most widely used is called albuterol, of which there are many brands. A second, less commonly used rescue medicine is called levalbuterol. Both are used to help relax the airway muscles, allowing the airway to open up and make it easier to breathe. The benefits are short-lived, typically lasting four hours or less.

The second group of medications is preventative medicines, of which there are many different forms, inhaled corticosteroids being the principle class. These medications are used on a daily basis to prevent an asthma attack from occurring.

Asthma medications can be thought of like sunburn medicines. **Preventative medications, like sun block, are to be used prior to the onset of wheezing and should be used on a daily basis to protect the lungs.** However, unlike sun block, should wheezing occur, many doctors will recommend to continue the preventative medicine(s) through the duration of the asthma exacerbation.

**Rescue medications, like aloe vera in the case of a sunburn, should be used once the wheezing has set in and relief is needed.** Like aloe vera, albuterol should be used as needed until the child is able to breathe normally again, after which the preventative medicine is needed once again to prevent another exacerbation.

Just as sun block cannot prevent every sunburn, preventative asthma medications will not prevent every asthma exacerbation. However, diligent use of preventative medications will significantly reduce the number of asthma episodes and help to prevent serious complications.

A doctor can help manage these medications and determine when they are needed, and when they can be stopped appropriately.

# TAKE-HOME POINTS

★ Sinus infections follow the same pathway as a middle ear infection.

★ Sinus infections are typically viral; most do not require antibiotics.

★ Bacterial pneumonias typically follow a cold, and are characterized by decreasing activity, increasing cough, and labored breathing.

★ Pinkeye is typically viral; most do not require antibiotics.

★ A bacterial pinkeye will produce discharge hourly and eventually produce redness and swelling of the skin surrounding the eye.

★ When a bacterial pinkeye is present, cheaper and older antibiotic eye drops will typically work just as well as new, "top-of-the-line" products.

★ Costochondritis and pleurisy are triggered by inflammation produced by a cold virus; both will improve with time and rest.

★ In genetically predisposed individuals, asthma can be triggered by a cold virus and may require medications to help control it.

Chapters 4, 5, and 6 explain the various ways in which a cold virus can lead to numerous complications in a child. Remember, there are two types of cold virus complications: inflammatory complications and clogging complications.

Depending on where in the respiratory tract a cold virus invades, it can manifest itself as rhinitis, a viral throat infection, a viral sinus infection, croup, laryngitis, bronchitis, bronchiolitis, or a viral pneumonia. If the cold virus moves outside of the respiratory tract, it can also trigger costochondritis, pleurisy or a viral pinkeye.

If enough mucus is produced by the cold virus and certain drainage pipes are clogged, an ear infection, a bacterial sinus infection, bacterial pneumonia, or bacterial pinkeye can also occur.

At times, several different complications may happen in succession, or even all together at once. Colds are the gateway infection to a host of unwanted conditions. Luckily, many of these conditions do not require antibiotics and will get better with time.

Finally, in those individuals with a genetic predisposition, the cold virus can also trigger an asthma attack. Thankfully, there are medications to help prevent and control asthma exacerbations.

A judicious doctor can help a family know when intervention is needed and when watchful waiting is best. Asthma medicines and antibiotics, when used appropriately, can help keep a child healthy, but it is important to use them only when truly needed.

What to Know Before Seeing Your Pediatrician

# Chapter 7

# GASTROENTERITIS (VOMITING AND DIARRHEA)

EVERY PARENT will, at some point, deal with a vomiting child. Watching your child empty the contents of their stomach can make anyone feel weak in the knees.

Thankfully, since most kids are now vaccinated against the rotavirus, it is unusual for them to become dehydrated to the point of requiring hospitalization. There are many viruses that can cause vomiting and diarrhea; however, rotavirus was one of the main culprits of serious cases necessitating hospitalization (worldwide, rotavirus is still a major threat in countries where the vaccine is not readily available).

Most kids suffering from gastroenteritis can recover at home with an orally administered rehydration technique (described later in the chapter) that is as effective as intravenous (IV) fluids given in an emergency room.

Although vomiting can happen for a number of reasons, the majority of cases will be the result of a stomach virus. Therefore, this chapter will focus on viral gastroenteritis (a.k.a. viral infections of the stomach and intestines).

## STOMACH VIRUSES DESTROY THE LINING OF THE GUT

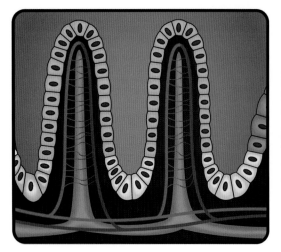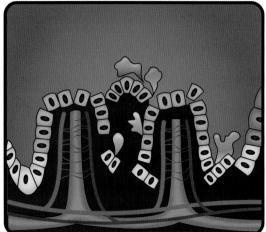

Like common cold viruses, stomach viruses destroy the body's tissues, specifically injuring the lining of the gut. The gut is populated throughout with structures called villi (which look like tiny mountains) that aid in the digestive process.

**The invading viruses destroy the intestinal villi, disrupting the digestive process and causing vomiting and diarrhea.** Once infected, the body will need time to recuperate and re-establish healthy gut villi.

Full recovery takes about two weeks, and diarrhea will often persist until the villi are restored. This will take time, and unfortunately, medications cannot accelerate the healing process.

What to Know Before Seeing Your Pediatrician

## TYPICAL TIMELINE OF A STOMACH VIRUS INFECTION

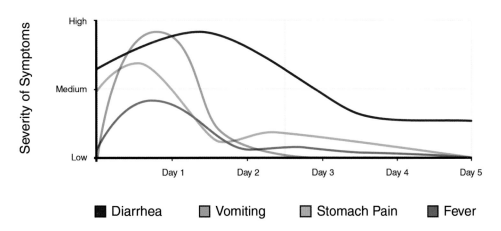

The typical timeline for a stomach virus is one to two days of vomiting, two to five days of fever and stomach pain, followed by one to two weeks of diarrhea.

**The biggest concern regarding a stomach virus is dehydration. The highest risk occurs during the first 48 hours of infection, when a child is losing fluids through both vomiting and diarrhea.**

Once the vomiting has passed, it is rare to become dehydrated from diarrhea alone, as long as fluids are readily available and consumed.

## THINK OF YOUR BODY AS A BOX OF WATER

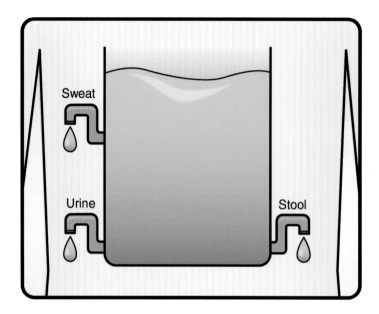

To understand how dehydration happens, imagine your body as a box of water. Fluids are inserted into the box by drinking throughout the day.

In a healthy individual, fluids are usually lost through sweating and urine (and a small amount through stool). **As long as the fluid taken in keeps up with the fluid lost, the body remains well-hydrated.**

What to Know Before Seeing Your Pediatrician

## VOMITING AND DIARRHEA INCREASE THE LOSS OF FLUIDS FROM THE BOX OF WATER

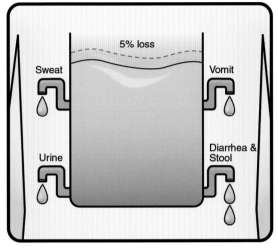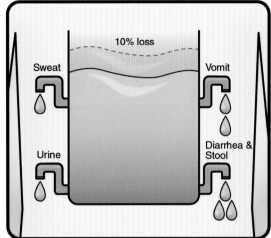

When a child becomes sick from a stomach virus, several things disrupt the box of water.

The child feels sick, leading to a decreased intake of fluids. The box also loses water faster than normal, as fluid escapes through vomiting and diarrhea in addition to its normal routes of loss.

In first world countries, it is unusual to see a child become dehydrated solely from diarrhea. Most cases of dehydration will happen when a child is vomiting six to eight times a day or more, and is unable to take in any fluids. Despite losing water through diarrhea, a child is usually able to drink enough fluids to offset what is lost as long as there is no vomiting.

**The likelihood and degree of dehydration is influenced by the frequency of vomiting and diarrhea, as well as the amount of fluid the child is able to take in.**

## SIGNS OF DEHYDRATION

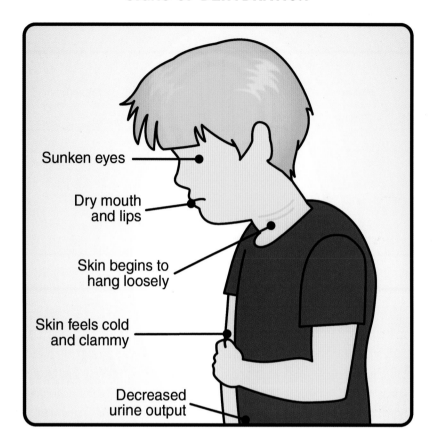

Sunken eyes

Dry mouth
and lips

Skin begins to
hang loosely

Skin feels cold
and clammy

Decreased
urine output

The signs of dehydration are as follows:

1. Noticeable decrease in activity level

2. Sunken eyes and sunken fontanelle (sunken soft spot—only seen in babies)

3. Dry mouth and lips (saliva becomes thick and gooey)

4. Decrease in skin turgor and skin hanging loosely

5. Cold and clammy skin

6. Decrease in urine output—child goes more than six to eight hours without urinating

As a child becomes dehydrated, many of the signs above will become apparent. A single sign of dehydration may not be cause for concern in and of itself.

**If multiple signs are apparent, especially if the child continues to vomit, a doctor**

What to Know Before Seeing Your Pediatrician

**should be seen to assess the hydration status and the need for possible IV fluids.** The younger the child is (particularly under 1 year of age) the less fluid reserve there is in the body; hence, there is greater risk for dehydration. For young kids, close monitoring is very important.

The oral hydration technique, discussed on the next page, can help prevent dehydration in most kids.

# REHYDRATION PROTOCOL

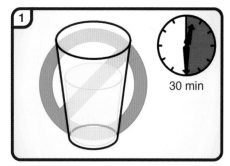

To allow stomach muscles to recuperate, do not give fluids for 30 minutes after vomiting.

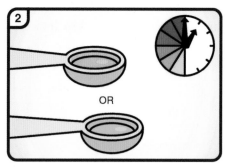

Give 1 teaspoon of oral rehydration solution (for children younger than 1 year old) or sports drink (for children older than 1 year) every five minutes for 30 minutes.

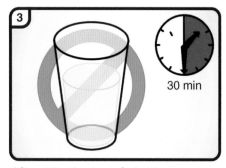

After 30 minutes of sipping every five minutes, wait an additional 30 minutes without drinking fluids. If they do not vomit, you can allow them to begin drinking oral rehydration solution or sports drink freely.

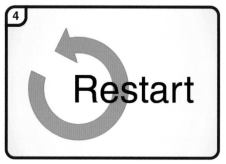

If at any time they vomit again, repeat the above cycle, starting from the beginning.

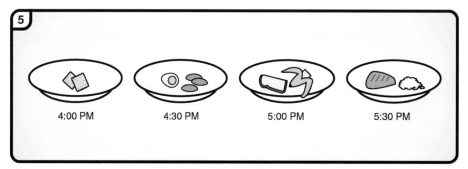

Advance diet slowly as your child demonstrates tolerance to fluids.

What to Know Before Seeing Your Pediatrician

The majority of stomach viruses can be handled at home by following the oral rehydration protocol. **After vomiting, the stomach needs time to recuperate. You do not want to immediately feed fluids to a vomiting child.** After a good 30-minute rest, small sips will help the stomach slowly tolerate fluids again. Once the stomach proves it can tolerate fluids, normal drinking can resume, with a slow progression to solid foods. Unfortunately, the child may still continue to vomit and become dehydrated, despite following the oral rehydration protocol. When this happens, certain medications may help to combat nausea and vomiting. Occasionally, IV hydration in the emergency room may also be necessary. A child with any signs of dehydration must be evaluated by a doctor as soon as possible.

# REFEEDING CHART FOLLOWING A STOMACH VIRUS

| FOODS | FOODS TO USE | FOODS TO AVOID |
|---|---|---|
| **Milk and milk products, supplements/formula** 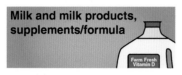 | 1% -2% milk or skim milk; low-fat yogurt after first 24 hours; lactose-free milk; all infant formulas | If lactose intolerance is suspected, avoid all regular milk and milk products temporarily |
| **Meat, poultry, fish, eggs, legumes, peanut butter, and cheese** 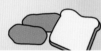 | Low-fat, grilled, or baked meat, fish, or poultry; low-fat cheese; boiled or poached eggs; any boiled or baked legumes with added fat; peanut butter in small amounts (<2 Tbsp) | High fat or fried meats, fish, poultry and/or cheese; fried eggs; peanut butter in large amounts (>2 Tbsp) |
| **Soups** 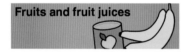 | Low-fat soups and broth | High fat creamed soups or chowders |
| **Breads, cereals, and starches** | Breads, cereals, rice, baked or mashed potatoes, pasta | Fried potatoes, French fries, doughnuts, muffins, chips; cereal with nuts, coconut, granola, wheat germ; bran cereals and muffins; popcorn |
| **Fruits and fruit juices** | Canned (packed in own juice) peaches, pears, applesauce, banana | Fruit juices |
| **Vegetables and vegetable juices** 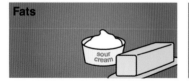 | All as tolerated | Vegetables cooked in butter, margarine, oils, or sauces |
| **Fats** | Minimal amounts of all fats; low-fat or fat free products such as salad dressing, sour cream, and cream cheese | Limit large amounts of all fats, including margarine, butter, oils, gravies, cream sauces, salad dressings, sour cream, cream cheese, etc. |
| **Desserts and sweets**  | Angel food cake, vanilla wafers, graham crackers, and other low-fat cookies, cakes, and desserts | Ice cream, sherbert, pies, popsicles, puddings, chocolate, and other high fat desserts |
| **Beverages**  | Sports drink, electrolyte solutions, e.g., oral rehydration solution | Regular soft drinks; caffeine containing drinks; fruit juices, high sugar containing drinks |
| **Miscellaneous**  | Spices, salt, mustard, ketchup, pickles in limited amounts | Highly seasoned foods; cream sauces; sugar, honey, jelly, syrup |

In the past, the BRAT diet (bananas, rice, applesauce, and toast) was the mainstay of refeeding a child who was recovering from a stomach virus. **Research has shown, however, that a more expansive diet will help the intestinal villi to recover sooner.** The faster the intestinal villi recover, the sooner digestion can return back to normal. As the child demonstrates their ability to tolerate fluids without vomiting, the refeeding chart can be utilized to select appropriate items to encourage solid food intake.

Recently, probiotics have become more mainstream. When given in sufficient quantity, probiotics may also help diarrhea to improve. Although the benefits of probiotics appear promising, research is still inconclusive. There are some mild risks with the use of probiotics, including becoming ill from the probiotic itself. A safe alternative would be to feed your child a plain yogurt that contains a high concentration of healthy bacteria.

## ANTI-DIARRHEAL MEDICATION CAN INCREASE THE RISK OF THE VIRUS SPREADING

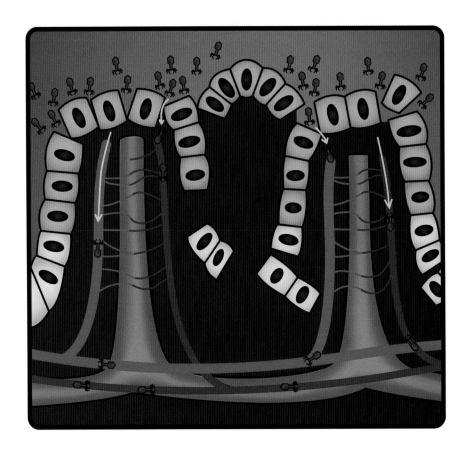

**Although there *are* anti-diarrheal medications available at the pharmacy, they are generally not recommended.** Peristalsis is the natural, forward wave-like movement of your intestines that works to properly expel waste products from your body after all the nutrition has been absorbed. Antidiarrheal medications work by slowing down the natural peristalsis movement of your intestines.

This simply masks the problem by forcing your body to hold the diarrhea longer, but does not promote any actual healing. **In fact, if you have gastroenteritis germs inside of you, getting them out of your system faster will help the recovery process.**

Anti-diarrheal medications simply delay the flushing out of the virus from the intestines. The longer the virus (or bacteria) stays in your intestines, the greater the likelihood is of the germ seeping into your blood vessels and spreading to other areas of your body, causing even more problems.

# ANTIBIOTICS SHOULD NOT BE USED
# FOR VOMITING/DIARRHEAL ILLNESSES

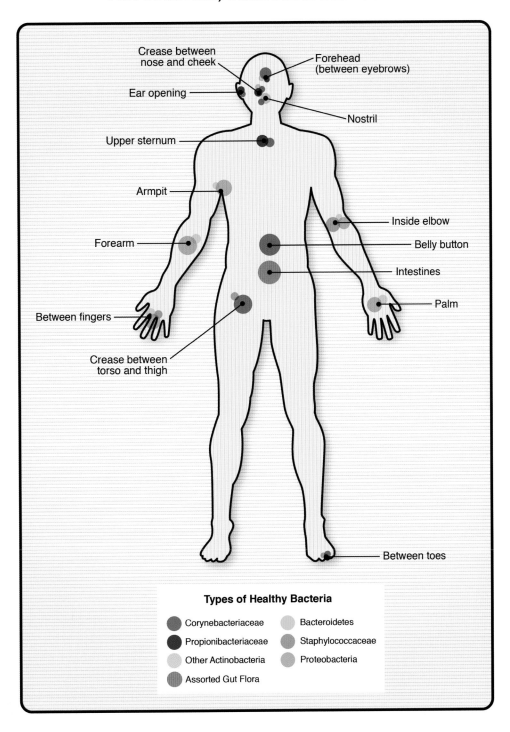

Hopefully by now it is clear that antibiotics do not help viral illnesses. Most vomiting/diarrheal illnesses are caused by viruses, yet some doctors still insist on prescribing antibiotics for diarrhea, due to the small percentage of cases caused by bacteria.

Although most bacterial illnesses should be treated with antibiotics, antibiotics are generally not recommended for a bacterial intestinal infection.

Remember that your body has healthy bacteria in your intestines that aid in the digestive process. **When antibiotics are taken, the good bacteria get destroyed along with the bad bacteria. In the long run, this can slow down the recovery process.**

**What to Know Before Seeing Your Pediatrician**

## GASTROPARESIS AFTER A STOMACH VIRUS MAY DISRUPT THE NORMAL PERISTALSIS PROCESS

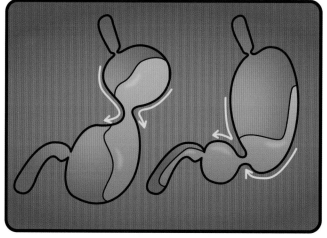

Normal Peristalsis

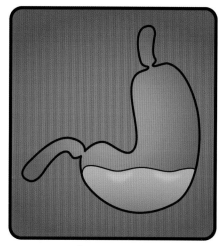

Gastroparesis

A small percentage of children will have vomiting that persists longer than two days, or which recurs a few days after the initial bout of vomiting has stopped.

The stomach and intestines normally push food through the digestive tract through a muscular wave called peristalsis. **Like any other muscle, if the stomach and intestines become tired from, or even injured by a virus, they may not function as efficiently.**

This stomach fatigue is called gastroparesis. When peristalsis no longer works properly and the stomach muscles are tired, food will not be pushed forward normally and will remain trapped in the stomach, which can lead to recurrent episodes of vomiting.

As with the initial bout of gastroenteritis, the biggest thing to watch out for with gastroparesis is dehydration. The activity level of the child and urine output should be monitored to ensure a child is not losing too many fluids.

If there is any concern for dehydration, a proper evaluation by the child's doctor can determine whether IV fluids or hospitalization might be necessary. Most cases of gastroparesis will resolve with time and a proper oral hydration regimen.

# SIGNS OF SERIOUS ISSUES WHEN VOMITING

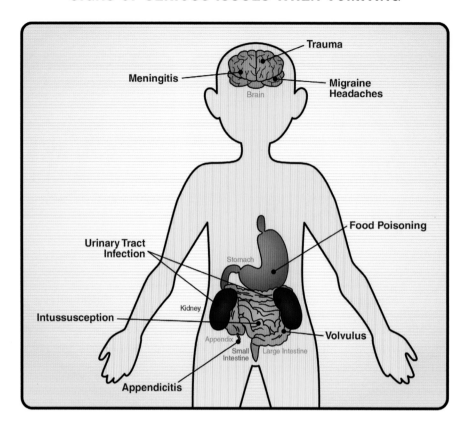

Not every case of vomiting will be caused by a stomach virus. **Depending on the symptoms, the doctor may need to rule out other causes of vomiting which may be more serious than a simple stomach virus, and which could require immediate intervention.**

Reasons to have the child evaluated promptly by a doctor are listed below:

1. Vomiting green bile (bile with a fluorescent, greenish-yellow tinge)
2. Vomiting blood
3. Blood in diarrhea
4. Vomiting six or more times in a 24-hour period
5. Significant abdominal pain, especially in the lower right side of the abdomen
6. Significant lethargy
7. Significant irritability
8. Pain when urinating or foul-smelling urine

What to Know Before Seeing Your Pediatrician

# AIRING OUT THE DIAPER AREA CAN HELP PREVENT A RASH

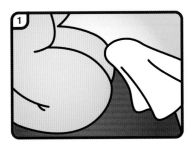 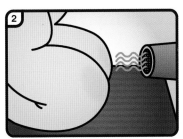 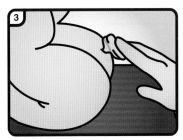

After stooling, clean the diaper area with warm water or chemical-free wipes

Air the diaper area out for five minutes or use a blow dryer on a cool setting to thoroughly dry the area

Apply a thick coating of diaper rash cream or petroleum jelly after drying

One of the common side effects from diarrhea is a diaper rash. Diarrhea is watery and typically acidic, which can irritate the skin.

A diaper rash is difficult to cure until the diarrhea fully resolves. Parents can help control the rash by following the above protocol. If you use a blow dryer to air out the diaper area, be sure to put it on the cool setting to avoid harming the baby. **As the diarrhea fades, so will the diaper rash.**

If the skin appears to be breaking down or the rash is worsening despite following the protocol shown above, a visit to the doctor may be necessary.

## CANDIDA (FUNGAL) DIAPER RASH

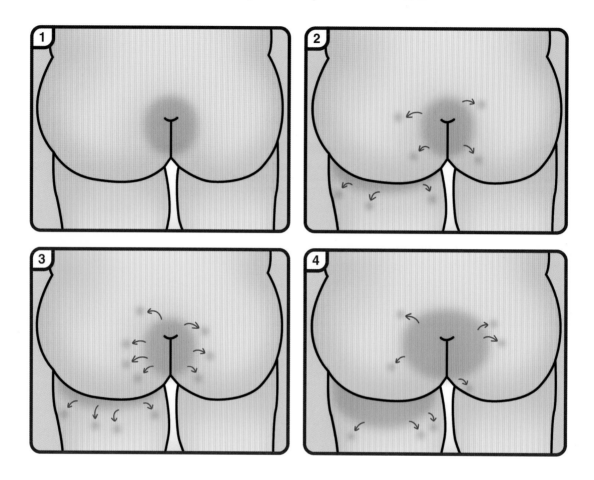

At times, after a diaper rash sets in, an infection of the diaper area triggered by a fungus called candida can further complicate the rash.

Unlike a simple diaper rash, where the acidity of the stool irritates the skin, a candida rash is an actual infection that spreads over time until appropriately treated with an anti-fungal cream.

There are two signs that help distinguish a candida diaper rash from a simple diaper rash. The first is the presence of the diaper rash in the creases of the skin. Fungus will typically affect the creases, whereas a simple irritation rash will not.

Second is the presence of satellite lesions surrounding the diaper rash. **The candida rash will grow in size by shooting out small satellite lesions from the central base.** The satellite lesions will then grow and eventually meld with the central base, expanding the size of the rash over time.

# TAKE-HOME POINTS

★ Stomach viruses destroy gut villi, which need time to recuperate.

★ Vomiting typically lasts one to two days; diarrhea typically lasts one to two weeks.

★ Think of your body as a "box of water" in which the input needs to keep up with the output.

★ Do not use anti-diarrheal medications, as they can prolong the illness.

★ Do not use antibiotics. They do not treat viruses and can destroy healthy gut bacteria.

★ Oral rehydration, when done correctly, is as effective as IV fluids in an emergency room.

★ Gastroparesis (fatigue of the gastrointestinal muscles) can prolong vomiting episodes.

★ Airing out the diaper area can help prevent/control a diaper rash caused by diarrhea.

★ Involvement of the creases and the presence of satellite lesions may be signs of a candida diaper rash, which will require anti-fungal cream.

★ Vomiting can be serious, and certain signs warrant an evaluation by a doctor.

Vomiting and diarrhea will happen throughout childhood, but it is the rare case wherein a child will require more than oral rehydration to fully recover. With a simple oral rehydration technique, most cases of stomach viruses can be observed at home.

The main goal with any stomach virus is to keep the child hydrated appropriately so that the "box of water" does not lose more water than it takes in.

Luckily, while vomiting can appear dangerous, most children will recover quickly with supportive measures.

## Chapter 8

# RETURNING TO SCHOOL AFTER A SICKNESS

**A**FTER ENSURING that your child is getting better from a sickness, the next thing to figure out is when to send them back to school.

Understanding how germs are spread and the science behind contagiousness can help parents and schools minimize lost school and work days, while protecting other kids from getting sick unnecessarily.

An ideal school policy is designed to prevent outbreaks of serious illness, while maximizing the educational opportunities for all children. Aggressive quarantining will only minimally prevent common illnesses from spreading, as most colds and stomach viruses are ubiquitous and plentiful. Unfortunately, return-to-school-rules tend to err on the side of being overly restrictive, without any proven research or science backing their policies.

Children's play groups also tend to have a code of "unwritten rules," most of which are not scientifically based. When navigating these waters, many are guided more by old wives tales and individual nuances than scientific facts.

In general, children with mild symptoms, such as a cough, runny nose, and infrequent diarrhea should be allowed to return to school and be around other children as long as they have the energy to make it through the planned activities.

With most run-of-the-mill viruses, the small number of benefits to be found in quarantining sick children to reduce the transmission of germs is far outweighed by the educational benefits of having kids return to school.

## YOU CAN BE CONTAGIOUS WITH A GERM BEFORE, DURING, AND AFTER AN ILLNESS

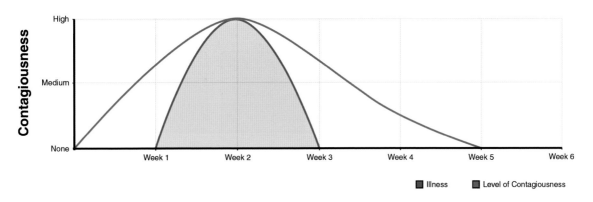

It would be easier to prevent the spread of germs if sick-appearing people were the only spreaders of the germs.

**However, you will be spreading germs *before* you are actually sick, *while* you are coming down with an illness, and even *after* you fully recover, regardless of whether or not you display any symptoms.**

Sometimes, the body will shed the offending germ for weeks, even after becoming completely healthy. This is why it is impossible for even the most careful parent and cautious school policy to prevent the spread of germs.

This is not to say that nothing can be done. Good hygiene habits, such as washing hands and covering one's mouth with an elbow when coughing, are probably the best way to reduce the spread of germs throughout the school. But while the spread of germs can be reduced, it cannot be fully eliminated.

## THE MORE SECRETIONS YOU HAVE, THE MORE CONTAGIOUS YOU ARE

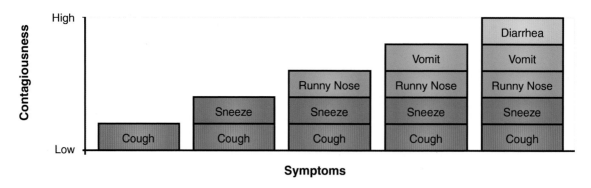

In general, you are most contagious when you are actually feeling sick. Droplets of fluid expressed from the body act as vessels for the germs, carrying them toward the next victim.

**The more fluids secreting out of your body (such as mucus, vomit, eye boogers, drool, diarrhea, or saliva), the more contagious you are.** Secretions will typically peak as the illness peaks, but remember that germs are still shed (though in lesser quantities) before and after the child actually feels sick.

What to Know Before Seeing Your Pediatrician

# BRIEF SUMMARY OF AAP GUIDELINES FOR WHEN TO STAY HOME

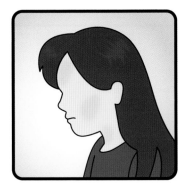 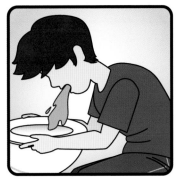 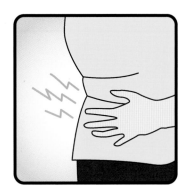

Some germs are more serious than others. Germs such as the cold virus; stomach virus; and hand, foot and mouth disease are very common. In general, these viruses are not that serious, and are so commonplace that even the strictest quarantining policy cannot prevent their spread. All children will catch these common viruses multiple times throughout the first few years of life.

But other germs are less common, more serious in consequence, and usually more controllable (from a public health standpoint), and therefore demand stricter policies.

**The American Academy of Pediatrics (AAP) has written detailed guidelines to help parents and schools know when a child should stay home. The following is an abbreviated list of symptoms, any of which warrant staying home and/or seeing the doctor:**

- Fever, when accompanied by behavior changes or other symptoms such as sore throat, rash, vomiting, diarrhea, earache, etc.

- Diarrhea (frequent, runny, watery stools); more than two stools above the baseline number of stools per day or if the diaper cannot contain the diarrhea.

- Blood in the stool not explained by dietary change, medication, or hard stool.

- Vomiting two or more times in a 24-hour period.

- Body rash with fever.

- Sore throat with fever and swollen glands or mouth sores with drooling.

- Severe coughing, with the child getting red or blue in the face or making a high-pitched whooping sound after coughing.

- Persistent abdominal pain (more than two hours) or intermittent pain with other signs and symptoms.

- Signs of possible severe illness, such as irritability, unusual tiredness, or neediness that compromises caregivers' ability to care for others.

- Uncontrolled coughing or wheezing, continuous crying, or difficulty breathing.

**What to Know Before Seeing Your Pediatrician**

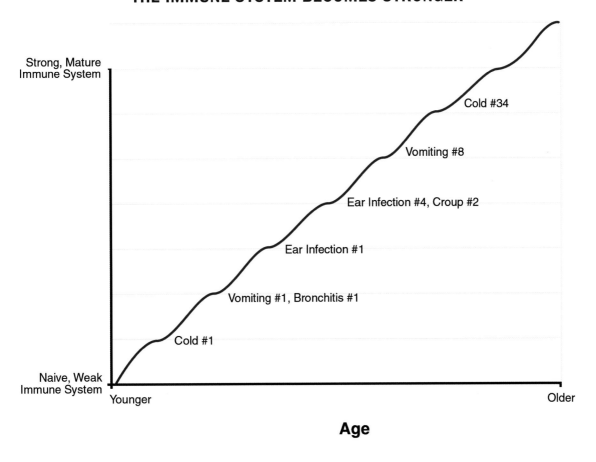

## AS THE BODY ENCOUNTERS MORE GERMS, THE IMMUNE SYSTEM BECOMES STRONGER

Strong, Mature Immune System

Cold #34

Vomiting #8

Ear Infection #4, Croup #2

Ear Infection #1

Vomiting #1, Bronchitis #1

Cold #1

Naive, Weak Immune System

Younger

Older

**Age**

Even if you *could* prevent every sickness your child could catch, you probably shouldn't. Your child's immune system is a complex interaction of multiple components that work to keep their body healthy.

**Like a group of soldiers going through basic training, the immune system can only get stronger and wiser as it fights battles and matures along the way.**

An under-activated immune system will suffer from a lack of experience, which can lead to serious consequences. Research continues to show that an under-activated immune system may get bored and eventually go a little haywire, increasing the risk for other problems, such as autoimmune diseases (when the immune system turns on its own body) and allergies.

# TAKE-HOME POINTS

★ Children are typically contagious before, during, and after an illness.

★ The more bodily fluids being secreted, the more contagious you are.

★ Common germs are ubiquitous, making quarantining of these germs impossible.

★ The AAP guidelines can help determine whether or not a child needs to be quarantined.

★ Challenging the immune system makes it stronger, and may help prevent unwanted future risks such as autoimmune diseases and allergies.

Knowing when to send a child back to school requires good communication amongst the parent, the school, and the doctor.

Using guidelines published by the AAP can help determine whether quarantining a child at home is necessary.

The goal is to protect the public health at large from outbreaks of serious illnesses while maximizing school attendance for the child, and minimizing lost work days for the parent.

# Conclusion

A S MUCH as I love all of my patients and families (and hopefully they love me!), I know that they would rather be resting at home with family than sitting in my exam room.

Nothing can replace a good relationship between a family and their doctor, but I hope this book will encourage better communication and strengthen an already existing bond.

The goal of this book has been to equip you with some basic pediatric knowledge and concepts that will make future discussions with your doctor more fruitful and enlightening. It might even save you a few unnecessary visits to the office—and possibly some co-pays!

There *will* be times when a doctor and a prescription are necessary, but more often than not, all a sick child needs to recover is a little time and some tender loving care under the watchful eye of their parents.

# About the Author

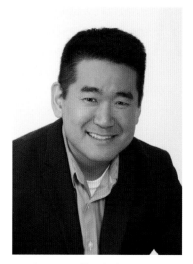

PETER JUNG was born in Passaic, New Jersey, in 1973 but has resided in Houston, Texas, for most of his life. He eagerly followed his father's footsteps into pediatrics, and after receiving his board certification in pediatrics and becoming a Fellow of the American Academy of Pediatrics in 2002, Dr. Jung went into private practice with his father. When his father retired in 2004, Dr. Jung opened the doors to Blue Fish Pediatrics. Today, Blue Fish Pediatrics has grown to include 13 providers in three Houston-area locations.

Dr. Jung is an Assistant Professor of Pediatrics at the University of Texas Medical School at Houston, and enjoys teaching pediatric residents, medical students, and nursing students at his community clinic year round. He has written for several local magazines, has been interviewed by local and national news programs about pediatric issues, and has taught several pediatric classes geared toward equipping parents.

Dr. Jung is active in his community at New Life Fellowship Baptist Church, where he leads the drama team and teaches the youth group. In his free time he enjoys basketball, softball, fishing, and spending time with his family.

Peter Y. Jung, M.D., F.A.A.P.
Rice University, Biology, 1995
Baylor College of Medicine, 1999
Ben Taub General Hospital and Texas Children's Hospital, Pediatric Residency, 2002
Blue Fish Pediatrics, Memorial Hermann Hospital System, 2005

# About the Illustrator

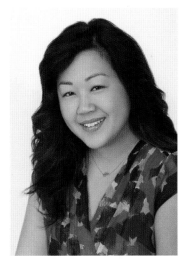

**B**ECKY SEO KIM was born in Mountain View, California, and has lived in both California and Texas for equal parts of her life (which she is very proud of).

In 2005, she graduated with a Bachelor of Arts in Visual Communication from American Intercontinental University, and has worked in marketing and as a graphic designer for most of her career. Becky's portfolio includes websites, digital ads, and menus for restaurants such as Popeye's, Fuddruckers, and Simply Seoul Kitchen. During her time with Woodlands Church, her work was distributed on an international level, ranging from booklets to brochures to sermon series artwork. She was also the lead designer for Woodlands Seminary, which launched in January 2015. This is Becky's first book illustration project, and she enjoys doing freelance design on top of her full-time job as an administrative and marketing coordinator.

Becky enjoys cooking and trying new restaurants, writing, playing video games, daydreaming about home improvement projects, and getting involved in her local church. Becky, her husband Sam, and their pit bull mix, Ernest, currently live in Houston.